Evidence-based Implant Dentistry
and Systemic Conditions

Evidence-based Implant Dentistry and Systemic Conditions

Fawad Javed, BDS, PhD

Department of General Dentistry
Eastman Institute for Oral Health
University of Rochester
Rochester, NY, USA

Georgios E. Romanos, DDS, PhD, Prof. Dr. med. dent.

Department of Periodontology
School of Dental Medicine
Stony Brook University
Stony Brook, NY, USA
&
Department of Oral Surgery and Implant Dentistry
School of Dentistry
Johann Wolfgang Goethe University
Frankfurt, Germany

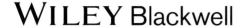

WILEY Blackwell

Registered Office
John Wiley & Sons, Inc., 111 River Street, Hoboken, NJ 07030, USA

Editorial Office
111 River Street, Hoboken, NJ 07030, USA

For details of our global editorial offices, customer services, and more information about Wiley products visit us at www.wiley.com.

Wiley also publishes its books in a variety of electronic formats and by print-on-demand. Some content that appears in standard print versions of this book may not be available in other formats.

Library of Congress Cataloging-in-Publication Data

Names: Javed, Fawad, 1976– author. | Romanos, Georgios, author.
Title: Evidence-based implant dentistry and systemic conditions / by Fawad Javed,
    Georgios E. Romanos.
Description: Hoboken, NJ : John Wiley & Sons, Inc., [2018] | Includes bibliographical
    references and index. |
Identifiers: LCCN 2018014591 (print) | LCCN 2018014780 (ebook) | ISBN 9781119212256 (pdf) |
    ISBN 9781119212263 (epub) | ISBN 9781119212249 (hardback)
Subjects: | MESH: Dental Implants | Evidence-Based Dentistry | Risk Factors
Classification: LCC RK667.I45 (ebook) | LCC RK667.I45 (print) | NLM WU 640 | DDC 617.6/93–dc23
LC record available at https://lccn.loc.gov/2018014591

Cover Design: Wiley
Cover Image: (top row images) © Dittmar May;
(middle and bottom row images) © Georgios E. Romanos

Set in 10/12pt Warnock by SPi Global, Pondicherry, India

Printed and bound in Singapore by Markono Print Media Pte Ltd

10 9 8 7 6 5 4 3 2 1

"I dedicate this book to my beloved wife, Dr. Hameeda Bashir Ahmed, and children, Sara Fawad and Rayan Fawad, for their endless love and support."

Fawad Javed

"To the love of my life, my partner in life adventures, my wife, Enisa, and our sweet little girl, our best creation, Stella Romanos."

Georgios E. Romanos

Contents

Preface

The use of dental implants for the oral rehabilitation of partially and completely edentulous individuals is increasing. With advancements in modern implant dentistry, the use of dental implants is not restricted to medically healthy individuals. Studies have reported that dental implants can osseointegrate and remain esthetically and functionally stable for prolonged durations in medically compromised patients (such as patients with acquired immune deficiency syndrome and diabetes mellitus) in a manner similar to systemically healthy individuals.

The fundamental theme of this book, *Evidence-based Implant Dentistry and Systemic Conditions,* is to base the oral rehabilitation of complete and partial anodontia using dental implants in patients with systemic diseases. In this book, each chapter is dedicated to a specific medical condition and its impact on the success and survival of dental implants. Pathophysiology of systemic diseases and their impact on osseointegration and bone loss around dental implants is discussed. Moreover, besides systemic conditions, this book describes how oral diseases such as history of periodontitis and oral cancer may affect the success and survival of dental implants, as well as the influence of habits (such as tobacco smoking and smokeless tobacco) on the outcome of dental implant therapy. In addition, several clinical and radiographic illustrations have been provided in the chapters to detail related concepts.

All chapters have been inked after a careful review of original and review articles published in indexed medical and dental journals. Every chapter is carefully blended to be consistent in aims/objectives to provide a foreseeable outcome.

From a clinical standpoint, this book is expected to provide an overview of the expected outcome of dental implant therapy in medically challenged patients; however, it also opens doors for further research in implant dentistry. In this regard, this book can be beneficial for students, postgraduate residents, clinicians, and researchers in dental and medical sciences.

1

Introduction

For centuries, dental practitioners have relied on partial dentures, complete dentures, and fixed prosthesis (such as bridges) for the replacement of missing teeth. Dental implants have revolutionized modern clinical practice and are a contemporary substitute to such traditional fixed and removable dental prosthesis. It is well known that dental implants can osseointegrate and remain functionally and aesthetically stable over long durations in patients with missing teeth. Studies have reported high success and survival rates of dental implants in systemically healthy individuals; however, dental implant therapy has also been reported to be successful among patients with systemic disorders, such as diabetes mellitus and acquired immune deficiency syndrome (AIDS).

This book provides essential information on the osseointegration and survival of dental implants in medically challenged patients. In this book, we compiled studies from indexed databases (including PubMed, MEDLINE, ISI web of knowledge, Scopus, and EMBASE) with reference to their impact on the survival and success of dental implants. These studies have formulated into individual chapters focusing on specific focused questions and data has been presented using a systematic review approach. The content of this book is centered on evidence-based dental implant therapy among patients with systemic diseases. Moreover, each chapter discusses the outcomes of the respective studies and recommendations for future research are also presented.

Evidence-based Implant Dentistry and Systemic Conditions, First Edition.
Fawad Javed and Georgios E. Romanos.
© 2018 John Wiley & Sons, Inc. Published 2018 by John Wiley & Sons, Inc.

2

Evidence-Based Grading of Studies

This book follows an *evidence-based grading* approach in order to make judgments about quality of evidence and strength of the study/studies included in each chapter. This approach will give researchers, clinicians, and students a clear overview of the level of scientific evidence relating to each chapter. This grading system is based on the methodology adopted across studies.

Level of Evidence Grade

A Evidence from randomized controlled trials

B Evidence from at least one randomized controlled trial

C Evidence from at least one well designed case-control study

D Evidence from at least one well-designed clinical study that was not randomized

E No evidence

Evidence-based Implant Dentistry and Systemic Conditions, First Edition.
Fawad Javed and Georgios E. Romanos.

3

Dental Implants in Adult Patients with Autism Spectrum Disorders

Introduction

Autism spectrum disorder, or ASD, is a group of developmental disorders that includes a variety/spectrum of symptoms, skills, and levels of disability (Scott et al., 2017). Patients with ASD usually have these characteristics: (a) Ongoing social problems such as resistance to communication and interaction with others; (b) repetitive behaviors and limited interests or activities; (c) Symptoms that hurt an individuals' ability to function in various areas of life (Scott et al., 2017). The precise etiology of ASD remains unclear; however, a number of risk factors have been associated with the etiology of ASD. These include genetic factors (genetic differences associated with the X chromosome), neurobiological factors (problems with genetic code development involving multiple brain regions), and environmental factors (exposure to drugs and environmental toxicants) (Abrahams and Geschwind, 2010; Coe et al., 2012a; Coe et al., 2012b; Landrigan et al., 2012).

A compromised oral health status has been reported in adult patients with ASD. In a study from Sweden, dental caries and periodontal health status were assessed among 47 adults with ASD and 69 age- and gender-matched controls (Blomqvist et al., 2015). The results showed a significantly reduced stimulated salivary flow rate among patients with ASD as compared to controls. Buccal gingival recession was more often manifested in patients with ASD than controls (Blomqvist et al., 2015). Although there was no statistically significant difference in dental caries among patients with and without ASD, the authors hypothesized that adults with ASD are more susceptible to dental caries than healthy adults, most likely as a consequence of a reduced salivary flow rate in ASD adults (Blomqvist et al., 2015). However, in another study, a statistically significant association was reported between ASD and the prevalence of dental caries. Other oral manifestations among adults with ASD are bruxism, self-perpetrated oral lesions, and dental malocclusions (most commonly anterior open bite) (Orellana et al., 2012).

Materials and Methods

Focused Question

Can dental implants osseointegrate and remain functionally stable in patients with ASD?

Evidence-based Implant Dentistry and Systemic Conditions, First Edition.
Fawad Javed and Georgios E. Romanos.
© 2018 John Wiley & Sons, Inc. Published 2018 by John Wiley & Sons, Inc.

Eligibility Criteria

The following eligibility criteria were entailed: (a) Original studies; (b) clinical studies; (c) intervention: bone-to-implant contacts in patients with ASD; and (d) use of statistical methods. Letters to the editor, historic reviews, commentaries, case-reports, and articles published in languages other than English were not sought.

Literature Search Strategy

To address the focused question, PubMed/MEDLINE (National Library of Medicine, Washington DC) and Google-Scholar databases were searched up to February 2018 using different combinations of the following key words: "autism," "bone-to-implant contact," "osseointegration," "implant," "survival," and "success." Reference lists of potentially relevant original and review articles were hand searched to identify studies that could have been missed during the initial search. Any disagreement between the authors regarding study selection was resolved by discussion. The pattern of the present systematic review was customized to primarily summarize the pertinent data.

A vigilant review of indexed literature revealed no studies that assessed the success and survival of dental implants in adults with ASD (Table 3.1).

Table 3.1 Success and/or survival rate of dental implants in adult patients with autism spectrum disorders.

Authors et al.	Age	Gender	Implant success/survival rate	Conclusion
There are no studies in indexed literature.				

Conclusion
There are no studies in indexed literature that have assessed whether dental implants can osseointegrate and remain functionally stable in patients with ASD. Hence, further studies are warranted in this regard.
GRADE ACCORDING TO LEVEL OF EVIDENCE: **E**

References

Abrahams, B. S. and Geschwind, D. H. 2010. Connecting genes to brain in the autism spectrum disorders. *Archives of Neurology* 67, pp. 395–399.

Blomqvist, M., Bejerot, S. and Dahllof, G. 2015. A cross-sectional study on oral health and dental care in intellectually able adults with autism spectrum disorder. *BMC Oral Health* 15, pp. 81.

Coe, B. P., Girirajan, S. and Eichler, E. E. 2012a. A genetic model for neurodevelopmental disease. *Current Opinion in Neurobiology* 22, pp. 829–836.

Coe, B. P., Girirajan, S. and Eichler, E. E. 2012b. The genetic variability and commonality of neurodevelopmental disease. *American Journal of Medical Genetics. Part C, Seminars in Medical Genetics* 160c, pp. 118–129.

Landrigan, P. J., Lambertini, L. and Birnbaum, L. S. 2012. A research strategy to discover the environmental causes of autism and neurodevelopmental disabilities. *Environmental Health Perspectives* 120, pp. a258–260.

Orellana, L. M., Silvestre, F. J., Martinez-Sanchis, S., Martinez-Mihi, V. and Bautista, D. 2012. Oral manifestations in a group of adults with autism spectrum disorder. *Medicina Oral, Patologia Oral y Cirugia Bucal* 17, pp. e415–419.

Scott, M., Jacob, A., Hendrie, D., Parsons, R., Girdler, S., Falkmer, T. and Falkmer, M. 2017. Employers' perception of the costs and the benefits of hiring individuals with autism spectrum disorder in open employment in Australia. *PloS one* 12, pp. e0177607.

4

Dental Implants in Patients with Cardiovascular Disorders

Introduction

Cardiovascular diseases (CVD) are a group of diseases that include atherosclerosis, congestive heart failure, coronary artery disease, hypertension, and vascular stenosis. It has been proposed that restricted supply of oxygen and nutrients to tissues may negatively affect osseointegration in patients with CVD (Elsubeihi and Zarb, 2002). To our knowledge from indexed literature, only a limited number of studies have assessed the influence of CVD on osseointegration of dental implants (Khadivi et al., 1999). It has been reported that the risk of stroke is 80% higher for nonsmoking patients with up to 24 teeth as compared to individuals who had 25 or more teeth (Joshipura et al., 2003). Likewise, results from another study reported an association to exist between periodontitis and increased risk of ischemic stroke compared with patients without periodontitis, gingivitis, or tooth loss (Wu et al., 2000).

The correlation between periodontitis and CVD has several possible pathophysiologic links. An increased systemic burden of bacteria, endotoxin, and other bacterial products could induce an abundant production of proinflammatory cytokines, cause inflammatory cell proliferation into large arteries, and increase the production of clotting factors (such as fibrinogen) through the liver, which may contribute to atherogenesis and thromboembolic events (Carroll and Sebor, 1980; Mask, 2000). Moreover, periodontopathogenic microbes may induce platelet aggregation that may be thrombogenic when entering the systemic circulation as in periodontitis (Herzberg and Weyer, 1996; 1998). Furthermore, bacterial toxins (lipopolysaccharides) may also damage the endothelial cells by attacking the arterial lining (Reidy and Bowyer, 1977). These results indicate that there is a relationship between periodontitis and CVD.

Since a previous history of periodontitis is a significant risk factor for peri-implant diseases (Romanos et al., 2015), it is hypothesized the outcome of dental implant therapy is compromised in patients with CVD compared with systemically healthy controls.

Objective

The aim of this chapter is to review indexed literature to determine whether dental implants can osseointegrate and remain functionally stable in adult patients with CVD.

Evidence-based Implant Dentistry and Systemic Conditions, First Edition.
Fawad Javed and Georgios E. Romanos.
© 2018 John Wiley & Sons, Inc. Published 2018 by John Wiley & Sons, Inc.

Materials and Methods

Focused Question

The addressed focused question was, "Can dental implants osseointegrate and remain functionally stable in adult patients with CVD?"

Eligibility Criteria

The following eligibility criteria were entailed: (a) Clinical studies and (b) placement and survival of dental implants in adult patients with CVD. Literature reviews, letters to the editor, commentaries, and articles published in languages other than English were excluded.

Literature Search

PubMed/Medline (National Library of Medicine, Bethesda, Maryland), EMBASE, ISI-Web of Knowledge, SCOPUS, and Google-Scholar databases were searched up to and including June 2016 using the following key words in different combinations: "dental implant," "cardiovascular diseases," "osseointegration," "heart attack," "ischemic heart disease," "coronary heart disease," "angina pectoris," "atherosclerosis," "stroke," "survival," and "success." Titles and abstracts of studies that fulfilled the eligibility criteria were screened and checked for agreement. Full texts of studies judged by title and abstract to be relevant were read and assessed in accordance with the eligibility criteria (as stated above). In addition, hand searching of the reference lists of potentially relevant original and review studies was also performed and checked for agreement via discussion.

Results

Results from a retrospective analysis of patients with certain types of CVD showed no statistically significant difference in the implant failure rates among patients with and without CVD (Khadivi et al., 1999). This study concluded that patients with controlled CVD are not at an increased risk of failure of osseointegration (Khadivi et al., 1999).

In another retrospective study, influence of CVD on implant failure, up to one week after the second stage of surgery was evaluated (van Steenberghe et al., 2002). The results showed that there was no statistically significant association between CVD and failure of osseointegration (van Steenberghe et al., 2002). Similarly, in the study by Alsaadi and associates, CVD were not associated with an increased incidence of early implant failures (Alsaadi et al., 2007). In another retrospective analysis, the authors reported that CVD such as hypertension and ischemic heart diseases are not significantly associated with early implant loss (Alsaadi et al., 2008). Although results from a publication showed that a history CVD is associated with dental implant failure (Neves et al., 2016); it has also been reported that oral rehabilitation with dental implants among patients with or without CVD is a valid treatment (Nobre Mde et al., 2016) (Table 4.1).

Discussion

The literature search revealed that there is a dearth of studies assessing the long-term success/survival of dental implants in patients with CVD. However, the results indicate that as long as CVD is controlled (via therapeutic strategies such as medication), it is not a contraindication to dental implant therapy.

Table 4.1 Outcome of assessing the outcome of implant therapy among patients with cardiovascular diseases.

Authors et al.	Study design	Participants	Outcome
Khadivi et al. (1999)	Retrospective	Group 1: 39 patients with CVD Group 2: 98 without CVD	There was no difference in implant survival rates among patients with and without controlled CVD.
van Steenberghe et al. (2002)	Prospective	399[†]	CVD was not associated with implant failure.
Alsaadi et al. (2007)	Retrospective	2004[†]	CVD was not associated with implant failure.
Alsaadi et al. (2008)	Retrospective	283[†]	CVD was not associated with implant failure.
Neves et al. (2016)	Retrospective	721[†]	CVD was not associated with implant failure.
Nobre Mde et al. (2016)	Retrospective	Group 1: 38 patients with CVD Group 2: 32 without CVD	CVD was not associated with implant failure.

CVD: cardiovascular diseases
[†]Patients had systemic diseases, including CVD. The exact number of patients with CVD remained unknown.

Conclusion
From the literature reviewed, it seems that dental implants can osseointegrate and remain functionally stable in patients with CVD; however, further long-term follow-up studies are needed in this regard. GRADE ACCORDING TO LEVEL OF EVIDENCE: **D**

References

Alsaadi, G., Quirynen, M., Komarek, A. and van Steenberghe, D. 2007. Impact of local and systemic factors on the incidence of oral implant failures, up to abutment connection. *Journal of Clinical Periodontology* 34, pp. 610–617. doi:10.1111/j.1600-051X.2007.01077.x.

Alsaadi, G., Quirynen, M., Michiles, K., Teughels, W., Komarek, A. and van Steenberghe, D. 2008. Impact of local and systemic factors on the incidence of failures up to abutment connection with modified surface oral implants. *Journal of Clinical Periodontology* 35, pp. 51–57. doi:10.1111/j.1600-051X.2007.01165.x.

Carroll, G. C. and Sebor, R. J. 1980. Dental flossing and its relationship to transient bacteremia. *Journal of Periodontology* 51, pp. 691–692. doi:10.1902/jop.1980.51.12.691.

Elsubeihi, E. S. and Zarb, G. A. 2002. Implant prosthodontics in medically challenged patients: the University of Toronto experience. *Journal of Canadian Dental Association* 68, pp. 103–108.

Herzberg, M. C. and Meyer, M. W. 1996. Effects of oral flora on platelets: possible consequences in cardiovascular disease. *Journal of Periodontology* 67, pp. 1138–1142. doi:10.1902/jop.1996.67.10s.1138.

Herzberg, M. C. and Weyer, M. W. 1998. Dental plaque, platelets, and cardiovascular diseases. *Annals of Periodontology* 3, pp. 151–160. doi:10.1902/annals.1998.3.1.151.

Joshipura, K. J., Hung, H. C., Rimm, E. B., Willett, W. C. and Ascherio, A. 2003. Periodontal disease, tooth loss, and incidence of ischemic stroke. *Stroke* 34, pp. 47–52.

Khadivi, V., Anderson, J. and Zarb, G. A. 1999. Cardiovascular disease and treatment outcomes with osseointegration surgery. *Journal of Prosthetic Dentistry* 81, 533–536.

Mask, A. G., Jr. (2000). Medical management of the patient with cardiovascular disease. *Periodontol* 2000 23, pp. 136–141.

Neves, J., de Araujo Nobre, M., Oliveira, P., Martins Dos Santos, J. and Malo, P. 2016. Risk Factors for Implant Failure and Peri-Implant Pathology in Systemic Compromised Patients. *Journal of Periodontology*. doi:10.1111/jopr.12508.

Nobre Mde, A., Malo, P., Goncalves, Y., Sabas, A. and Salvado, F. 2016. Outcome of dental implants in diabetic patients with and without cardiovascular disease: A 5-year post-loading retrospective study. *European Journal of Oral Implantology* 9, pp. 87–95.

Reidy, M. A. and Bowyer, D. E. 1977. Scanning electron microscopy: Morphology of aortic endothelium following injury by endotoxin and during subsequent repair. *Atherosclerosis* 26, pp. 319–328.

Romanos, G. E., Javed, F., Delgado-Ruiz, R. A. and Calvo-Guirado, J. L. 2015. Peri-implant diseases: a review of treatment interventions. *Dental Clinics of North America* 59, pp. 157–178. doi:10.1016/j.cden.2014.08.002.

van Steenberghe, D., Jacobs, R., Desnyder, M., Maffei, G. and Quirynen, M. 2002. The relative impact of local and endogenous patient-related factors on implant failure up to the abutment stage. *Clinical Oral Implants Research* 13, pp. 617–622.

Wu, T., Trevisan, M., Genco, R. J., Dorn, J. P., Falkner, K. L. and Sempos, C. T. 2000. Periodontal disease and risk of cerebrovascular disease: the first national health and nutrition examination survey and its follow-up study. *Archives of Internal Medicine* 160, pp. 2749–2755.

5

Dental Implants in Patients with Crohn's Disease

Introduction

What Is Crohn's Disease?

Crohn's disease (CD) is an idiopathic chronic inflammatory disorder of the gastrointestinal tract, which may also affect the oral cavity (Scheper and Brand, 2002). CD is characterized by the presence of several antibody-antigen complexes, leading to autoimmune inflammatory processes in many parts of the body – for example, enteritis, recurrent oral ulceration, vasculitis, arthritis, or keratoconjunctivitis.

Global Incidence/Prevalence of Crohn's Disease

Increasing trends in the incidence and prevalence of CD have been reported almost globally, with Canada, France, Italy, New Zealand, Scotland, and Scandinavia being among the most distinct regions (Economou and Pappas, 2008; Galeone et al., 2017). In the United States, there are 400,000 to 600,000 patients with CD. In the US state of Minnesota, an incidence rate of $7/10^5$ has been reported or CD (Jess et al., 2006). Early reports from Canada (Quebec and Ontario) have shown a lower incidence and prevalence of CD ($0.7/10^5$ and $33/10^5$, respectively) (Hiatt and Kaufman, 1988; Economou and Pappas, 2008). An Australian study conducted between the years 1971 and 2001 showed an increase in annual rates from 0.13 to $2/10^5$ in a typical urban patient population (Phavichitr et al., 2003). Although the incidence of CD remains low in Asian countries (including China, India, and Malaysia), cases of CD are often misdiagnosed as enteric tuberculosis or amebic colitis (Desai and Gupte, 2005; Zheng et al., 2005; Hilmi and Wang, 2006; Economou and Pappas, 2008). Therefore, the Asian continent may also harbor a vast majority of CD patients worldwide.

Oral Health Status in Patients with Crohn's Disease

The prevalence rates of oral manifestations in patients with CD vary between 5% to 20%; however, in pediatric patients, the prevalence is much higher (48% to 80%) (Orosz and Sonkodi, 2004). It has been reported that patients with CD perceive their oral health to be worse than individuals without CD (controls) (Rikardsson et al., 2009). In this study, oral health–related problems, such as gingivitis and dental caries, were more often reported by patients with CD than controls (Rikardsson et al., 2009).

Evidence-based Implant Dentistry and Systemic Conditions, First Edition.
Fawad Javed and Georgios E. Romanos.
© 2018 John Wiley & Sons, Inc. Published 2018 by John Wiley & Sons, Inc.

In addition, clinical scores of the markers of periodontitis (bleeding on probing, probing pocket depth, clinical attachment loss) have been reported to be higher in patients with CD than controls (Vavricka et al., 2013). Furthermore, ulcerative lesions involving the lips, tongue, buccal mucosa, and posterior pharynx have also been reported in patients with CD as compared to controls (Estrin and Hughes, 1985).

Hypothesis

Since CD is associated with nutritional and immune defects (Hwang and Wang, 2007), it is hypothesized that CD increases the risk of early implant failure.

Objective

The aim of this chapter is to review indexed literature to determine whether dental implants can osseointegrate and remain functionally stable in patients with CD.

Results

Five studies were included (van Steenberghe et al., 2002; Alsaadi et al., 2007; Alsaadi et al., 2008a; Alsaadi et al., 2008b; Peron et al., 2015). Four studies reported that CD is significant factor for implant (van Steenberghe et al., 2002; Alsaadi et al., 2007; Alsaadi et al., 2008a; Alsaadi et al., 2008b). In a retrospective study by van Steenberghe et al. (2002) two of three patients with CD had implant failures (3 out of 10 inserted implants failed). In their study, Peron et al. (2015) reported two cases with CD in whom dental implants successfully osseointegrated and remained functionally stable up to 13 and 12 months of follow-up (Table 5.1).

Discussion

There is a scarcity of literature regarding the stability and long-term survival of dental implants in patients with CD. Four studies were identified that showed that CD was significantly associated with early implant failure. It has been speculated that the presence of antigen-antibody complexes in patients with CD may be held responsible for autoimmune inflammatory processes in several parts of the body (such as enteritis, vasculitis, recurrent oral ulceration, arthritis, or kerato-conjunctivitis), including the bone-implant interface (van Steenberghe et al., 2002). In addition, malnutrition encountered in patients with CD may also cause deficient bone healing around the implant (Esposito et al., 1998). However, the role of other factors such as claustrophobia, smoking, and poor bone quantity that may also negatively influence bone-to-implant interface and jeopardize implant success and/or survival cannot be disregarded.

In the study by Alsaadi et al. (2007), CD was significantly associated with early implant failure and exhibited an odds ratio (OR) of 7.95 (95% CI of 3.47 to 18.24), the highest OR of all systemic factors evaluated in the study. However, it is pertinent to mention that the authors did not provide the number of patients with CD treated or the number of implant

Table 5.1 Assessment of osseointegration and survival of dental implants in patients with Crohn's disease.

Authors et al. (Year)	Study design	Patients with Crohn's disease (n)	Mean age of patients with Crohn's disease	Duration of Crohn's disease (in years)	Number of implants failed/placed (n)	Jaw location	Duration of follow-up	Outcome
van Steenberghe et al. (2002)	Retrospective	3*	NA	NA	3/10	NA	~6 months	CD was significantly associated with early implant failure.
Alsaadi et al. (2007)[+]	Retrospective	NA	NA	NA	NA	NA	NA	CD was significantly associated with early implant failure.
Alsaadi et al. (2008a)[+]	Retrospective	NA	NA	NA	NA	NA	2 years	CD was significantly associated with early implant failure.
Alsaadi et al. (2008b)[+]	Retrospective	NA	NA	NA	NA	NA	NA	CD was significantly associated with early implant failure.
Peron et al. (2015)	Case-series	2	35-year-old male	~13 years	None	Maxilla	13 months	The implant replacing maxillary left first premolar was functionally and esthetically stable.
			36-year-old female	~10 years	None	Maxilla	12 months	The implant replacing maxillary left first premolar was functionally and esthetically stable.

NA: Not available

*The total population comprised of 399 individuals (including 3 patients with Crohn's disease).

[+]This study only reported the mean age patients with trauma. Since no significant difference in age was reported among participants of the population assessed in this study, it is assumed that patients with Crohn's disease belonged to the same age group.

failures in these patients. Furthermore, from the literature reviewed, it was observed that the study population comprised patients with various systemic disorders, one of which was CD. Nevertheless, all studies reported a prognosis of dental implants in patients with CD. The only study that showed positive outcome of dental implant therapy in patients with CD was by Peron et al. (2015). In this study, trabecular metal implants were placed in the regions of missing maxillary premolars in two patients with CD. At approximately 1 year of follow-up, the implants were esthetically and functionally stable in both patients (Peron et al., 2015). Moreover, crestal bone heights between baseline and the following year of follow-up showed no statistically significant difference in both patients. This is most likely associated with the microgrooved collar design of trabecular metal implants (Peron et al., 2015).

Further studies on patients with CD with a larger patient population are needed to assess the osseointegration and long-term survival of dental implants in these patients.

Conclusion
There is insufficient evidence to assess whether dental implants can remain functionally stable in patients with CD. Hence, further studies are warranted in this regard.
GRADE ACCORDING TO LEVEL OF EVIDENCE: **D**

References

Alsaadi, G., Quirynen, M., Komarek, A. and van Steenberghe, D. 2007. Impact of local and systemic factors on the incidence of oral implant failures, up to abutment connection. *Journal of Clinical Periodontology* 34, pp. 610–617. doi:10.1111/j.1600-051X.2007.01077.x.

Alsaadi, G., Quirynen, M., Komarek, A. and van Steenberghe, D. 2008a. Impact of local and systemic factors on the incidence of late oral implant loss. *Clinical Oral Implants Research* 19, pp. 670–676. doi:10.1111/j.1600-0501.2008.01534.x.

Alsaadi, G., Quirynen, M., Michiles, K., Teughels, W., Komarek, A. and van Steenberghe, D. 2008b. Impact of local and systemic factors on the incidence of failures up to abutment connection with modified surface oral implants. *Journal of Clinical Periodontology* 35, pp. 51–57. doi:10.1111/j.1600-051X.2007.01165.x.

Desai, H. G. and Gupte, P. A. 2005. Increasing incidence of Crohn's disease in India: is it related to improved sanitation? *Indian Journal of Gastroenterology* 24, pp. 23–24.

Economou, M. and Pappas, G. 2008. New global map of Crohn's disease: Genetic, environmental, and socioeconomic correlations. *Inflammatory Bowel Diseases* 14, pp. 709–720. doi:10.1002/ibd.20352.

Esposito, M., Hirsch, J. M., Lekholm, U. and Thomsen, P. 1998. Biological factors contributing to failures of osseointegrated oral implants. (II). Etiopathogenesis. *European Journal of Oral Science* 106, pp. 721–764.

Estrin, H. M. and Hughes, R. W., Jr. 1985. Oral manifestations in Crohn's disease: report of a case. *American Journal of Gastroenterology* 80, pp. 352–354.

Galeone, C., Pelucchi, C., Barbera, G., Citterio, C., La Vecchia, C. and Franchi, A. 2017. *Crohn's disease in* Italy: A critical review of the literature using different data sources. *Digest of Liver Disease.* doi:10.1016/j.dld.2016.12.033.

Hiatt, R. A. and Kaufman, L. 1988. Epidemiology of inflammatory bowel disease in a defined northern California population. *The Western Journal of Medicine* 149, pp. 541–546.

Hilmi, I., Tan, Y. M. and Goh, K. L. 2006. Crohn's disease in adults: observations in a multiracial Asian population. *World Journal of Gastroenterology* 12, pp. 1435–1438.

Hwang, D. and Wang, H. L. 2007. Medical contraindications to implant therapy: Part II: Relative contraindications. *Implant Dentistry* 16, pp. 13–23. doi:10.1097/ID.0b013e31803276c8.

Jess, T., Loftus, E. V., Jr., Harmsen, W. S., Zinsmeister, A. R., Tremaine, W. J., Melton, L. J., III, Munkholm, P. and Sandborn, W. J. 2006. Survival and cause specific mortality in patients with inflammatory bowel disease: a long term outcome study in Olmsted County, Minnesota, 1940-2004. *Gut* 55, pp. 1248–1254. doi:10.1136/gut.2005.079350.

Orosz, M. & Sonkodi, I. 2004. [Oral manifestations in Crohn's disease and dental management]. *Fogorv Sz* 97, pp. 113–117.

Peron, C., Javed, F. and Romanos, G. E. 2015. Crohn's Disease and Trabecular Metal Implants: A report of two clinical cases and literature review. *Journal of Osseointegration* 7, pp. 52–56.

Phavichitr, N., Cameron, D. J. and Catto-Smith, A. G. 2003. Increasing incidence of Crohn's disease in Victorian children. *Journal of Gastroenterology and Hepatology* 18, pp. 329–332.

Rikardsson, S., Jonsson, J., Hultin, M., Gustafsson, A. and Johannsen, A. 2009. Perceived oral health in patients with Crohn's disease. *Oral Health and Preventive Dentistry* 7, pp. 277–282.

Scheper, H. J. and Brand, H. S. (2002). Oral aspects of Crohn's disease. *International Dental Journal* 52, pp. 163–172.

van Steenberghe, D., Jacobs, R., Desnyder, M., Maffei, G. and Quirynen, M. 2002. The relative impact of local and endogenous patient-related factors on implant failure up to the abutment stage. *Clinical Oral Implants Research* 13, pp. 617–622.

Vavricka, S. R., Manser, C. N., Hediger, S., Vogelin, M., Scharl, M., Biedermann, L., Rogler, S., Seibold, F., Sanderink, R., Attin, T., Schoepfer, A., Fried, M., Rogler, G. and Frei, P. 2013. Periodontitis and gingivitis in inflammatory bowel disease: a case-control study. *Inflammatory Bowel Diseases* 19, pp. 2768–2777. doi:10.1097/01.MIB.0000438356.84263.3b.

Zheng, J. J., Zhu, X. S., Huangfu, Z., Gao, Z. X., Guo, Z. R. and Wang, Z. 2005. Crohn's disease in mainland China: a systematic analysis of 50 years of research. *Chinese Journal of Digestive Diseases* 6, pp. 175–181. doi:10.1111/j.1443-9573.2005.00227.x.

6

Dental Implants in Patients with Eating Disorders

Introduction

What Are Eating Disorders?

Eating disorders (EDs) are abnormal eating habits, which may involve either insufficient or excessive food consumption thereby jeopardizing an individual's physical and/or mental health status (Bell et al., 2017).

Types and Prevalence of Eating Disorders

The most common forms of EDs include anorexia nervosa (AN) and bulimia nervosa (BN) (Fischer et al., 2014; Tortorella et al., 2014). AN is characterized by malnutrition and restricted food consumption (Romanos et al., 2012; Swinbourne et al., 2012); and BN is characterized by excessive food consumption (binge eating), followed by inappropriate compensatory behaviors such as self-induced vomiting, use of laxatives, and excessive exercise (Romanos et al., 2012; Swinbourne et al., 2012). In general, EDs are a heterogeneous combination of AN- and BN-like EDs (Johansson et al., 2012).

Only a few studies have reported the prevalence of EDs (Garner and Garfinkel, 1980; Preti et al., 2009; Smink et al., 2014). EDs are a major health issue among children and adolescents of all ethnic groups in the United States (Nicholls and Viner, 2005). According to the American Dietetic Association (2001), EDs are dominant among adolescent females with prevalence rates of up to 5%. In Europe, lifetime estimated prevalence of 0.48%, 0.51%, 1.12%, 0.72%, and 2.15% have been reported for AN, BN, binge-eating disorder, sub-threshold binge-eating disorder, and any binge eating, respectively (Preti et al., 2009). These values are up to eight times higher in females as compared to males with EDs (Preti et al., 2009). In a recent cohort study, prevalence of AN, BN, and binge-eating disorders were reported to be 1.7%, 0.8%, and 2.3%, respectively, among Dutch females (Smink et al., 2014). In this study (Smink et al., 2014), EDs were relatively rare among males.

Oro-Dental Status in Patients with Eating Disorders

Dental erosions, dry and/or cracked lips, and burning-tongue syndrome are common manifestations in patients with EDs as compared to individuals without EDs (controls) (Johansson et al., 2012; Romanos et al., 2012). Moreover, signs and symptoms of temporomandibular disorders, including dizziness, facial pain, headache, jaw tiredness, tongue thrusting and lump feeling in the throat, concentration difficulties, and sleep disturbances are also

Evidence-based Implant Dentistry and Systemic Conditions, First Edition.
Fawad Javed and Georgios E. Romanos.
© 2018 John Wiley & Sons, Inc. Published 2018 by John Wiley & Sons, Inc.

frequently in patients with EDs (Johansson et al., 2012; Romanos et al., 2012). Furthermore, patients with EDs undergoing dental treatments (under local anesthesia) have been reported to display greater levels of dental fear and anxiety than those without EDs (Sirin et al., 2011).

Objective

Since oro-dental status is compromised in patients with EDs, the aim of this chapter is to review indexed literature to determine whether dental implants can osseointegrate and remain functionally stable in patients with EDs.

Materials and Methods

Eligibility Criteria

The following eligibility criteria were entailed: (a) clinical studies and (b) placement and survival of dental implants in patients with EDs. Literature reviews, letters to the editor, and commentaries were excluded.

Literature Search

PubMed/Medline (National Library of Medicine, Bethesda, Maryland), EMBASE, ISI-Web of Knowledge, SCOPUS, and Google-Scholar databases were searched through February 2018 using the following key words in different combinations: "eating disorder," "anorexia nervosa," "bulimia nervosa," "dental implant," "binge eating," "osseointegration," "survival," and "success." Titles and abstracts of studies that fulfilled the eligibility criteria were screened and checked for agreement. Full texts of studies judged by title and abstract to be relevant were read and assessed in accordance with the eligibility criteria (as stated above). In addition, hand searching of the reference lists of potentially relevant original and review studies was also performed and checked for agreement via discussion.

Results

Following an exhaustive search of indexed literature, 13 studies were initially identified. Twelve studies, which did not fulfill the eligibility criteria, were excluded (Table 6.1). Therefore, one case-report was included and processed for data extraction (Ambard and Mueninghoff, 2002). In this case-report, oral rehabilitation using dental implants was performed in a 31-year-old nonsmoking female with a 10-year history of BN (Ambard and Mueninghoff, 2002). Clinical examination showed multiple crowns with extensive cervical caries, and prognosis of all teeth was poor. Peri-implant tissues were inflamed and lack of keratinized tissue necessitated additional periodontal procedures before a definitive restoration could be placed in this patient.

Most of the remaining teeth were endodontically treated. According to the treatment plan, these teeth were extracted and followed by implant placement and fixed restorations. The goal of the prosthetic plan was to provide first molar occlusion to the patient using eight maxillary and six mandibular implants. The one-year follow-up results

Table 6.1 Characteristics and outcome of the study that assessed osseointegration and survival of dental implants in a patient with eating disorders.

Authors et al. (Year)	Study design	Age of patient (in years)	Type of eating disorder	Duration of eating disorder (in years)	Number of implants placed (n)	Jaw location	Duration of follow-up (in months)	Outcome
Ambard and Mueninghoff (2002)	Case-report	31	Bulimia Nervosa	10	14	Maxilla (8 implants) Mandible (6 implants)	12	● Implants were aesthetically and functionally stable. ● Patients' self-esteem had also improved.

showed that the implants were aesthetically and functionally stable. The patients' self-esteem had also improved at follow-up (Ambard and Mueninghoff, 2002).

Discussion

It is speculated that placement and long-term survival of dental implants with a history of EDs may challenge clinicians. However, to our knowledge from indexed literature, there is insufficient evidence to verify whether dental implants can osseointegrate and remain functionally stable in patients with EDs. Results from an *in-vitro* study showed that exposure of implant surfaces to a simulated vomit solution (pH 3.8) did not significantly affect the implant surface characteristics (such as roughness) (Matsou et al., 2011). This study concluded that regurgitation of the acidic gastric contents in the mouth of bulimic patients does not influence the implant surface characteristics (Matsou et al., 2011), which suggests that dental implants can safely be placed in patients with BN. It is hypothesized that chronic regurgitation of acidic gastric components into the oral cavity impair soft tissue healing around newly placed in patients with EDs. Moreover, it is imperative for oral healthcare providers to be aware of the oral manifestations of EDs, as some of these patients may prefer not to disclose their medical history (particularly that of AN or BN).

In the study by Ambard and Mueninghoff (2002), implants placed in a bulimic patient were functionally stable after one year of follow-up. However, it is noteworthy that the self-esteem of this patient had also improved following implant placement. This is indicative of the fact that patients with EDs, who are potential candidates for future dental implant therapy, should be referred to healthcare professionals for adjunct psychological therapy. An improved self-esteem in patients with EDs may respond well to dental implant therapy as compared to those with low self-esteem. However, further long-term prospective studies are warranted in this regard.

Conclusion
To date, there is insufficient evidence to determine whether dental implants can remain functionally stable in patients with EDs. Hence, further studies are warranted in this regard. GRADE ACCORDING TO LEVEL OF EVIDENCE: **D**

References

2001. Position of the American Dietetic Association: nutrition intervention in the treatment of anorexia nervosa, bulimia nervosa, and eating disorders not otherwise specified (EDNOS). *Journal of the American Dietetic Association* 101, pp. 810–819.

Ambard, A. and Mueninghoff, L. 2002. Rehabilitation of a bulimic patient using endosteal implants. *Journal of Prosthodontics* 11, pp. 176–180.

Bell, C., Waller, G., Shafran, R. and Delgadillo, J. 2017. Is there an optimal length of psychological treatment for eating disorder pathology? *International Journal of Eating Disorders*. doi:10.1002/eat.22660.

Fischer, S., Meyer, A. H., Dremmel, D., Schlup, B. and Munsch, S. 2014. Short-term cognitive-behavioral therapy for binge eating disorder: long-term efficacy and predictors of long-term treatment success. *Behaviour Research and Therapy* 58C, pp. 36–42. doi:10.1016/j.brat.2014.04.007.

Garner, D. M. and Garfinkel, P. E. 1980. Socio-cultural factors in the development of anorexia nervosa. *Psychological Medicine* 10, pp. 647–656.

Johansson, A. K., Norring, C., Unell, L. and Johansson, A. 2012. Eating disorders and oral health: a matched case-control study. *European Journal of Oral Science* 120, pp. 61–68. doi:10.1111/j.1600-0722.2011.00922.x.

Matsou, E., Vouroutzis, N., Kontonasaki, E., Paraskevopoulos, K. M. and Koidis, P. 2011. Investigation of the influence of gastric acid on the surface roughness of ceramic materials of metal-ceramic restorations. *An in vitro study. The International Journal of Prosthodontics* 24, pp. 26–29.

Nicholls, D. and Viner, R. 2005. Eating disorders and weight problems. *British Medical Journal* 330, pp. 950–953. doi:10.1136/bmj.330.7497.950.

Preti, A., Girolamo, G., Vilagut, G., Alonso, J., Graaf, R., Bruffaerts, R., Demyttenaere, K., Pinto-Meza, A., Haro, J. M. and Morosini, P. 2009. The epidemiology of eating disorders in six European countries: results of the ESEMeD-WMH project. *Journal of Psychiatric Research* 43, pp. 1125–1132. doi:10.1016/j.jpsychires.2009.04.003.

Romanos, G. E., Javed, F., Romanos, E. B. and Williams, R. C. 2012. Oro-facial manifestations in patients with eating disorders. *Appetite* 59, pp. 499–504. doi:10.1016/j.appet.2012.06.016.

Sirin, Y., Yucel, B., Firat, D. and Husseinova-Sen, S. 2011. Assessment of dental fear and anxiety levels in eating disorder patients undergoing minor oral surgery. *Journal of Oral and Maxillofacial Surgery* 69, pp. 2078–2085. doi:10.1016/j.joms.2010.12.050.

Smink, F. R., van Hoeken, D., Oldehinkel, A. J. and Hoek, H. W. 2014. Prevalence and severity of DSM-5 eating disorders in a community cohort of adolescents. *International Journal of Eating Disorders*. doi:10.1002/eat.22316.

Swinbourne, J., Hunt, C., Abbott, M., Russell, J., St Clare, T. and Touyz, S. 2012. The comorbidity between eating disorders and anxiety disorders: prevalence in an eating disorder sample and anxiety disorder sample. *Australian & New Zealand Journal of Psychiatry* 46, pp. 118–131. doi:10.1177/0004867411432071.

Tortorella, A., Brambilla, F., Fabrazzo, M., Volpe, U., Monteleone, A. M., Mastromo, D. and Monteleone, P. 2014. Central and peripheral peptides regulating eating behaviour and energy homeostasis in anorexia nervosa and bulimia nervosa: a literature review. *European Eating Disorders Review*. doi:10.1002/erv.2303.

7

Dental Implants in Patients with Epilepsy

Introduction

What is Epilepsy?

Seizures are a common manifestation in epileptic patients. Epilepsy is defined as a transient occurrence of signs and/or symptoms due to abnormal excessive or synchronous neuronal activity in the brain (Fisher et al., 2014). This definition requires the occurrence of at least one epileptic seizure (Fisher et al., 2014). The electroencephalogram and magnetic resonance imaging are usually performed for the diagnosis of epilepsy (Morano et al., 2017).

Etiologic Classification of Epilepsy

It is worth mentioning that very few attempts have been made to synoptically list the causes of epilepsy. Previous classifications of epilepsy have largely focused on clinical manifestations of epilepsy (Kammerman and Wasserman, 2001); however, Shorvon (2011) proposed a scheme for a classification of epilepsy by etiology. According to this classification, epilepsy is classified into four subtypes (Shorvon, 2011):

1) *Idiopathic epilepsy:* epilepsy most likely of a genetic origin without any gross neuro-anatomic or neuropathologic anomaly.
2) *Symptomatic epilepsy:* epilepsy of an acquired or genetic etiology, associated with gross anatomic or pathologic abnormalities, and/or clinical features, indicative of underlying disease.
3) *Provoked epilepsy:* epilepsy in which a specific systemic or environmental factor is the principle cause of seizures with no gross causative neuroanatomic or neuropathologic changes.
4) *Cryptogenic epilepsy:* epilepsy of assumed symptomatic nature, in which the cause is unknown.

Global Prevalence of Epilepsy

Epilepsy is a common neurologic disorder, which affects nearly 50 million individuals worldwide. In developing countries, epilepsy has a prevalence of approximately 1%. In Western Europe, the age-adjusted prevalence of active epilepsy has been reported to be 5.4 per 1,000 individuals, with a higher prevalence in males as compared to females (Picot et al., 2008). In North America, more than 3 million individuals have epilepsy, and the overall epilepsy incidence is approximately 50 per 100,000 individuals per year (Theodore et al., 2006).

Evidence-based Implant Dentistry and Systemic Conditions, First Edition.
Fawad Javed and Georgios E. Romanos.
© 2018 John Wiley & Sons, Inc. Published 2018 by John Wiley & Sons, Inc.

Oral Health Status in Patients with Epilepsy

Gingival overgrowth (GO) is a common side of many anti-epileptic drugs (such as phenytoin). In a prospective study, GO was a common finding in 66 epileptic adults (mean age ~37 years) receiving phenytoin for more than one year (Lin et al., 2008). Likewise, in a recent study on 150 epileptic children, GO was reported as common side effect in 46% of the 12- to 17-year-old children on anti-epileptic drugs (Ghafoor et al., 2014). Furthermore, a case report also reported the occurrence of GO in a 60-year-old non–denture-wearing epileptic female, who was receiving phenytoin and phenobarbital drugs since 7 years old (Dhingra and Prakash, 2012).

Scores for decayed and missing teeth, loss of gingival attachment, dental plaque-index, and calculus-index have been reported to be significantly high in epileptic patients as compared to controls (Karolyhazy et al., 2003; Karolyhazy et al., 2005). According to Costa et al. (2014), patients with epilepsy are significantly more susceptible to poor oral hygiene, gingivitis, and periodontitis than controls. However, it has been reported that long term use of antiepileptic drugs (phenytoin and carbamazepine) does not result in increased risk for alveolar bone loss (Dahllof et al., 1993).

Hypothesis

Since epilepsy and GO are manageable and long-term use of antiepileptic drugs does not result in increased risk for alveolar bone loss (Dahllof et al., 1993; de Oliveira Guare et al., 2010; Baulac et al., 2014) in epileptic patients, it is hypothesized that dental implants can osseointegrate and remain functionally stable in epileptic patients.

Objective

The aim of this chapter is to review indexed literature to determine whether dental implants can osseointegrate and remain functionally stable in epileptic adult patients.

Materials and Methods

Eligibility Criteria

The following eligibility criteria were entailed: (a) clinical studies and (b) placement and survival of dental implants in epileptic adult patients. Literature reviews, letters to the editor, commentaries, and articles published in languages other than English were excluded.

Literature Search

PubMed/Medline (National Library of Medicine, Bethesda, Maryland), EMBASE, ISI-Web of Knowledge, SCOPUS, and Google-Scholar databases were searched through February 2018 using the following key words in different combinations: "dental implant," "epilepsy," "osseointegration," "seizure," "survival," and "success." Titles and abstracts of studies that fulfilled the eligibility criteria were screened and checked for agreement. Full texts of studies judged by title and abstract to be relevant were read and assessed in accordance with the eligibility criteria (as stated above). In addition, hand searching of the reference lists of potentially relevant original and review studies was also performed and checked for agreement via discussion.

Results

Following an exhaustive search of indexed literature, we found one retrospective study that assessed the osseointegration and survival of dental implants in patients with epilepsy (Cune et al., 2009). In this study, performance of endosseous dental implants was retrospectively assessed among patients with severe epilepsy and additional motor and/or intellectual impairments (Cune et al., 2009). A total of 134 implants were placed in 61 patients (~43 years old) and observed over a period of 16 years (Table 7.1). In general, clinical results showed mild inflammation of the peri-implant mucosa and an average peri-implant probing depth of 2 mm. There were no obvious signs of GO in the patient population. Periapical radiographs showed stable marginal bone levels. Three implants (in three different patients) failed during the observation period, demonstrating an estimated probability of functional implant survival of 97.6%. However, oral hygiene status was considered inadequate around 72% of the implants that were clinically examined ($n = 45$) (Cune et al., 2009). The primary results of this study are summarized in Table 7.2 (Cune et al., 2009).

Discussion

The literature search revealed that there is a dearth of studies assessing the osseointegration and long-term success/survival of dental implants in patients with seizures. The only study that was found in indexed literature was performed by Cune et al. (2009). In this study, peri-implant tissues showed mild inflammation, and the estimated probability of functional implant survival of implants was 97.6% (Cune et al., 2009). Despite the fact that, to date, this is the only evidence available in indexed literature, it is indicative that

Table 7.1 Implant data and number of patients included in survival statistics and clinical and radiologic investigations (modified from Cune et al. [2009]).

Total number of implants assessed in the study	134
Implants that were available for clinical examination	107
Implants that were clinically assessed	76
Implants available for radiologic examination	65
Implants that could not be radiologically assessed	11
Patients that were unavailable for follow-up	8
Uncooperative patients	6
Unloaded implants	4
Lost or failed implants	3
Patients who died after implant placement	10

Table 7.2 Characteristics and outcome of the study that assessed osseointegration and survival of dental implants in patients with epilepsy.

Authors et al. (Year)	Study design	Patients (n)	Mean age of patients (in years)	Duration of epilepsy (in years)	Number of implants placed (n)	Jaw location	Duration of follow-up (in years)	Outcome
Cune et al. (2009)	Retrospective	61	43.2 ± 14.9	10	134	Maxilla and Mandible	16	Three implants failed during the observation period, demonstrating an estimated probability of functional implant survival of 97.6%.

dental implants can osseointegrate and remain functionally stable in patients with seizures (epilepsy) (Cune et al. 2009). It is pertinent to mention that the nursing staff monitoring the patients included in the study by Cune et al. (2009) were educated about the significance of oral health and were also instructed to assure that the patients maintain a strict oral hygiene. In addition, in this study implants with ball-socket attachment were placed in edentulous patients to facilitate oral hygiene maintenance (Cune et al., 2009). Furthermore, in partially edentulous patients with anterior implants, the implant abutments were purposely weakened by grinding a transverse sleeve. This was done to allow the abutment to break in case of dental trauma or a seizure attack, thereby minimizing the possibility of any damage to the alveolar bone or the implant (Cune et al., 2009). Furthermore, since peri-implant bone levels remained stable in patients receiving antiepileptic drugs, it suggests that the use of antiepileptic drugs does not negatively influence alveolar bone levels around dental implants.

It is speculated that dental implants can osseointegrate and remain functionally stable in epileptic patients; however, further studies are needed to verify this hypothesis. It is recommended that epileptic patients who are selected for dental implant therapy be educated about the significance of oral hygiene maintenance with respect to the long-term stability and survival of implants. In addition, these patients should be instructed to strictly follow oral hygiene maintenance protocols and routinely visit their oral healthcare providers for follow-up.

Conclusion

There is insufficient evidence to determine whether dental implants can remain functionally stable in the long-term among patients with epilepsy. Hence, further studies are warranted in this regard.

GRADE ACCORDING TO LEVEL OF EVIDENCE: **D**

References

1981. Proposal for revised clinical and electroencephalographic classification of epileptic seizures. From the Commission on Classification and Terminology of the International League Against Epilepsy. *Epilepsia* 22, pp. 489–501.

Baulac, M., Patten, A. and Giorgi, L. 2014. Long-term safety and efficacy of zonisamide versus carbamazepine monotherapy for treatment of partial seizures in adults with newly diagnosed epilepsy: Results of a phase III, randomized, double-blind study. *Epilepsia*. doi:10.1111/epi.12749.

Costa, A. L., Yasuda, C. L., Shibasaki, W., Nahas-Scocate, A. C., de Freitas, C. F., Carvalho, P. E. and Cendes, F. 2014. The association between periodontal disease and seizure severity in refractory epilepsy patients. *Seizure* 23, pp. 227–230. doi:10.1016/j.seizure.2013.12.008.

Cune, M. S., Strooker, H., van der Reijden, W. A., de Putter, C., Laine, M. L. and Verhoeven, J. W. 2009. Dental implants in persons with severe epilepsy and multiple disabilities: a long-term retrospective study. *International Journal of Oral and Maxillofacial Implants* 24, pp. 534–540.

Dahllof, G., Preber, H., Eliasson, S., Ryden, H., Karsten, J. and Modeer, T. 1993. Periodontal condition of epileptic adults treated long-term with phenytoin or carbamazepine. *Epilepsia* 34, pp. 960–964.

de Oliveira Guare, R., Costa, S. C., Baeder, F., de Souza Merli, L. A. and Dos Santos, M. T. 2010. Drug-induced gingival enlargement: biofilm control and surgical therapy with gallium-aluminum-arsenide (GaAlAs) diode laser-A 2-year follow-up. *Special Care in Dentistry* 30, pp. 46–52. doi:10.1111/j.1754-4505.2009.00126.x.

Dhingra, K. and Prakash, S. 2012. Gingival overgrowth in partially edentulous ridges in an elderly female patient with epilepsy: a case report. *Gerodontology* 29, pp. e1201–1206. doi:10.1111/j.1741-2358.2012.00624.x.

Fisher, R. S., Acevedo, C., Arzimanoglou, A., Bogacz, A., Cross, J. H., Elger, C. E., Engel, J., Jr., Forsgren, L., French, J. A., Glynn, M., Hesdorffer, D. C., Lee, B. I., Mathern, G. W., Moshe, S. L., Perucca, E., Scheffer, I. E., Tomson, T., Watanabe, M. and Wiebe, S. 2014. ILAE official report: a practical clinical definition of epilepsy. *Epilepsia* 55, pp. 475–482. doi:10.1111/epi.12550.

Ghafoor, P. A., Rafeeq, M. and Dubey, A. 2014. Assessment of oral side effects of Antiepileptic drugs and traumatic oro-facial injuries encountered in Epileptic children. *Journal of International Oral Health* 6, pp. 126–128.

Kammerman, S. and Wasserman, L. 2001. Seizure disorders: Part 1. Classification and diagnosis. *Western Journal of Medicine* 175, pp. 99–103.

Karolyhazy, K., Kivovics, P., Fejerdy, P. and Aranyi, Z. 2005. Prosthodontic status and recommended care of patients with epilepsy. *Journal of Prosthetic Dentistry* 93, pp. 177–182. doi:10.1016/j.prosdent.2004.11.008.

Karolyhazy, K., Kovacs, E., Kivovics, P., Fejerdy, P. and Aranyi, Z. 2003. Dental status and oral health of patients with epilepsy: an epidemiologic study. *Epilepsia* 44, pp. 1103–1108.

Lin, C. J., Yen, M. F., Hu, O. Y., Lin, M. S., Hsiong, C. H., Hung, C. C. and Liou, H. H. 2008. Association of galactose single-point test levels and phenytoin metabolic polymorphisms with gingival hyperplasia in patients receiving long-term phenytoin therapy. *Pharmacotherapy* 28, pp. 35–41. doi:10.1592/phco.28.1.35.

Morano, A., Carni, M., Casciato, S., Vaudano, A. E., Fattouch, J., Fanella, M., Albini, M., Basili, L. M., Lucignani, G., Scapeccia, M., Tomassi, R., Di Castro, E., Colonnese, C., Giallonardo, A. T. and Di Bonaventura, C. 2017. Ictal EEG/fMRI study of vertiginous seizures. *Epilepsy Behavior* 68, pp. 51–56. doi:10.1016/j.yebeh.2016.12.031.

Picot, M. C., Baldy-Moulinier, M., Daures, J. P., Dujols, P. and Crespel, A. 2008. The prevalence of epilepsy and pharmacoresistant epilepsy in adults: a population-based study in a Western European country. *Epilepsia* 49, pp. 1230–1238. doi:10.1111/j.1528-1167.2008.01579.x.

Shorvon, S. D. 2011. The etiologic classification of epilepsy. *Epilepsia* 52, pp. 1052–1057. doi:10.1111/j.1528-1167.2011.03041.x.

Theodore, W. H., Spencer, S. S., Wiebe, S., Langfitt, J. T., Ali, A., Shafer, P. O., Berg, A. T. & Vickrey, B. G. 2006. Epilepsy in North America: a report prepared under the auspices of the global campaign against epilepsy, the International Bureau for Epilepsy, the International League Against Epilepsy, and the World Health Organization. *Epilepsia* 47, pp. 1700–1722. doi:10.1111/j.1528-1167.2006.00633.x.

8

Dental Implants in Patients with Hepatic Disorders

Introduction

Aspartate Aminotransferase

Aspartate aminotransferase (AST) is a pyridoxal phosphate-dependent transaminase enzyme, which plays an essential role in the metabolism of amino acids (Miura et al., 2017). AST is mainly found in the liver but is also present in other tissues, including the heart, red blood cells, and skeletal muscles. When body tissue or an organ such as the liver is diseased, additional AST is released into the bloodstream, thereby elevating its levels. In this regard, assessment of AST levels is commonly performed for the diagnosis of hepatic disorders (Pokorska-Spiewak et al., 2016; Miura et al., 2017).

Association between Aspartate Aminotransferase Activity and Periodontal and Peri-Implant Diseases

Elevated AST levels in the saliva and gingival crevicular fluid have been associated with periodontal inflammatory parameters (probing depth and gingival bleeding) (Fiorellini et al., 2000; Totan et al., 2006). It has been reported that salivary AST levels are significantly higher in patients with chronic periodontitis (CP) (Kudva et al., 2014); however, mechanical debridement of plaque and calculus from teeth surfaces results in a statistically significant decrease in salivary AST levels in patients with CP (Kudva et al., 2014). Similarly, increased AST activity in the peri-implant sulcular fluid, have been associated with peri-implant bleeding on probing and bone loss (Ruhling et al., 1999; Paolantonio et al., 2000).

Hypothesis

Since levels of AST in blood are significantly higher in patients with hepatic disorders and increased AST activity has been associated with periodontal and peri-implant diseases (Kudva et al., 2014), it is hypothesized that the outcomes of implant therapy are compromised in patients with hepatic disorders.

Evidence-based Implant Dentistry and Systemic Conditions, First Edition.
Fawad Javed and Georgios E. Romanos.
© 2018 John Wiley & Sons, Inc. Published 2018 by John Wiley & Sons, Inc.

Objective

The aim of this chapter is to review indexed literature to determine whether dental implants can remain functionally stable in patients with hepatic disorders.

Materials and Methods

Eligibility Criteria

The following eligibility criteria were entailed: (a) Clinical studies and (b) placement and survival of dental implants in animals or human patients with hepatic disorders. Literature reviews, letters to the editor, and commentaries were excluded.

Literature Search

PubMed/Medline (National Library of Medicine, Bethesda, Maryland), EMBASE, ISI-Web of Knowledge, SCOPUS, and Google-Scholar databases were searched up to February 2018 using the following key words in different combinations: "liver," "dental implant," "failure," "fibrosis," "hepatic," "hepatitis," "cirrhosis," "survival," "success." Titles and abstracts of studies that fulfilled the eligibility criteria were screened and checked for agreement. Full texts of studies judged by title and abstract to be relevant were read and assessed in accordance with the eligibility criteria (as already stated). In addition, hand searching of the reference lists of potentially relevant original and review studies was also performed and checked for agreement via discussion.

Results

There are no studies in indexed literature that assessed the success and survival rates of dental implants placed in patients with hepatic disorders (Table 8.1).

Table 8.1 Studies assessing the outcome of dental implant therapy among patients with hepatic disorders.

Authors et al. (Year)	Study design	Participants	Type of hepatic disorder	Implant success/ survival rate
There are no studies in indexed literature.				

Conclusion
There is no evidence to determine whether dental implants can remain functionally stable in patients with hepatic disorders. Hence, further studies are warranted in this regard. GRADE ACCORDING TO LEVEL OF EVIDENCE: **D**

References

Fiorellini, J. P., Nevins, M. L., Sekler, J., Chung, A. and Oringer, R. J. 2000. Correlation of peri-implant health and aspartate aminotransferase levels: a cross-sectional clinical study. *International Journal of Oral and Maxillofacial Implants* 15, pp. 500–504.

Kudva, P., Saini, N., Kudva, H. and Saini, V. 2014. To estimate salivary aspartate aminotransferase levels in chronic gingivitis and chronic periodontitis patients prior to and following non-surgical periodontal therapy: A clinico-biochemical study. *Journal of Indian Society of Periodontology* 18, pp. 53–58. doi:10.4103/0972-124x.128209.

Miura, Y., Kanda, T., Yasui, S., Takahashi, K., Haga, Y., Sasaki, R., Nakamura, M., Wu, S., Nakamoto, S., Arai, M., Nishizawa, T., Okamoto, H. and Yokosuka, O. 2017. Hepatitis A virus genotype IA-infected patient with marked elevation of aspartate aminotransferase levels. *Clinical Journal of Gastroenterology* 10, pp. 52–56. doi:10.1007/s12328-016-0700-5.

Paolantonio, M., Di Placido, G., Tumini, V., Di Stilio, M., Contento, A. and Spoto, G. 2000. Aspartate aminotransferase activity in crevicular fluid from dental implants. *Journal of Periodontology* 71, pp. 1151–1157. doi:10.1902/jop.2000.71.7.1151.

Pokorska-Spiewak, M., Kowalik-Mikolajewska, B., Aniszewska, M., Pluta, M., Walewska-Zielecka, B. and Marczynska, M. 2016. Predictors of liver disease severity in children with chronic hepatitis B. *Advances in Clinical and Experimental Medicine* 25, pp. 681–688. doi:10.17219/acem/60535.

Ruhling, A., Jepsen, S., Kocher, T. and Plagmann, H. C. 1999. Longitudinal evaluation of aspartate aminotransferase in the crevicular fluid of implants with bone loss and signs of progressive disease. *International Journal of Oral and Maxillofacial Implants* 14, pp. 428–435.

Totan, A., Greabu, M., Totan, C. and Spinu, T. 2006. Salivary aspartate aminotransferase, alanine aminotransferase and alkaline phosphatase: possible markers in periodontal diseases? *Clinical and Chemical Laboratory Medicine* 44, pp. 612–615. doi:10.1515/cclm.2006.096.

9

Dental Implants in Patients with Diabetes Mellitus

Introduction

Dental implants are a modern replacement to the conventional fixed and removable dental appliances. It is well known that systemic disorders, such as poorly controlled diabetes mellitus (DM), jeopardizes periodontal health and is also a significant risk factor for dental implant failure (Javed et al., 2007; Javed and Romanos, 2009; Oates et al., 2009). One explanation for this is that chronic hyperglycemia increases the formation and accumulation of glucose-mediated advanced glycation end products (AGEs) in the periodontal and systemic tissues in patients with poorly controlled DM (Holla et al., 2001; Murillo et al., 2008). These AGEs play a role in the pathogenesis and altered periodontal wound healing by activating the receptors for AGEs (RAGE) located on the periodontium (Holla et al., 2001). In addition, it has been reported that endothelial cells take up glucose passively in an insulin-independent manner, thereby causing tissue damage (Ebersole et al., 2008). Furthermore, chronic hyperglycemia has also been associated with alterations in host resistance by defective migration of polymorphonuclear leukocytes, impairment in phagocytosis and exaggeration in inflammatory response to microbial products (Soory, 2002). These factors may also be held responsible for the increase prevalence of peri-implant diseases (peri-implant mucositis and peri-implantitis) in patients with poorly controlled DM as compared to non-diabetic controls (Ferreira et al., 2006; Gomez-Moreno et al., 2014).

Optimal glycemic maintenance in patients diagnosed with DM has been reported to improve the overall health status (Mager et al., 2013). Studies have reported that dental implants and osseointegrate and remain functionally stable in patients with well-controlled DM in a manner contrast to patients with a poor metabolic control of DM (Kwon et al., 2005; Tawil et al., 2008; Lee et al., 2013). For example, in a clinical study by Tawil et al. (2008), implant survival rates were comparable among patients with well-controlled diabetes and nondiabetic controls. Likewise, in an experimental study, Casap et al. (2008) assessed the osseointegration of implant discs placed in tibial medullary spaces of 140 male diabetic and control rats. Histomorphometric results showed significantly higher trabecular bone volumes among controls and rats with well-controlled diabetes, as compared to those with poorly controlled diabetes. Similar results were reported by de Molon et al. (2013).

Since chronic hyperglycemia jeopardizes the outcome and survival rates of dental implants and glycemic maintenance enhances BIC in diabetic patients (McCracken et al., 2006; Casap et al., 2008; Inbarajan et al., 2012), it is tempting to speculate that well-controlled DM favors dental implant osseointegration in a manner similar to healthy

Evidence-based Implant Dentistry and Systemic Conditions, First Edition.
Fawad Javed and Georgios E. Romanos.
© 2018 John Wiley & Sons, Inc. Published 2018 by John Wiley & Sons, Inc.

individuals. The aim of this study, however, is to systematically review the effect of optimal glycemic control on the BIC in patients with DM.

Objective

The aim of this chapter is to assess indexed literature to determine whether dental implant can remain functionally stable in patients with diabetes mellitus.

Materials and Methods

Eligibility Criteria

The following eligibility criteria were entailed: (a) Original studies; (b) clinical and experimental studies; (c) intervention: BIC in patients/subjects with well-controlled DM; and (d) use of statistical methods. Letters to the editor, historic reviews, commentaries, case-reports, and articles published in languages other than English were not sought.

Literature Search

To address the focused question, PubMed/MEDLINE (National Library of Medicine, Washington DC) and Google-Scholar databases were searched through December 2016 using different combinations of the following key words: "diabetes mellitus," "bone to implant contact," "osseointegration," "implant," and "metabolic control." Titles and abstracts of studies obtained using this search strategy were screened by the authors (FJ and GER) and checked for agreement. Full texts of studies that were judged (by title and abstract) to be relevant were read and independently evaluated with reference to the eligibility criteria previously stated. Reference lists of potentially relevant original and review articles were hand searched to identify studies that could have been missed during the initial search. Any disagreement between the authors regarding study selection was resolved by discussion. The pattern of the present systematic review was customized to primarily summarize the pertinent data.

Results

Through the initial search, 35 studies were identified. Scrutiny of titles and full-texts of these studies reduced the number of articles to 17 (Shernoff et al., 1994; Balshi and Wolfinger, 1999; McCracken et al., 2000; Olson et al., 2000; Abdulwassie and Dhanrajani, 2002; Siqueira et al., 2003; Kopman et al., 2005; Kwon et al., 2005; McCracken et al., 2006; Casap et al., 2008; Tawil et al., 2008; Wang et al., 2011; Inbarajan et al., 2012; Malik et al., 2012; Lee et al., 2013; de Molon et al., 2013; Erdogan et al., 2014), which were processed for data extraction (Tables 9.1 and 9.2). Seventeen studies, which did not comply with the eligibility criteria, were excluded (see Appendix A). Out of the 18 studies (Shernoff et al., 1994; Balshi and Wolfinger, 1999; McCracken et al., 2000; Olson et al., 2000; Abdulwassie and Dhanrajani, 2002; Siqueira et al., 2003; Kopman et al., 2005; Kwon et al., 2005; McCracken et al., 2006; Casap et al., 2008; Tawil et al., 2008; Wang et al., 2011; Inbarajan et al., 2012; Malik et al., 2012; Lee et al., 2013; de Molon et al., 2013; Erdogan et al., 2014;

Table 9.1 Characteristics of clinical studies.

Authors et al.	Patient groups (n)	Mean age (in years)	Total implants inserted (n)	Duration of diabetes	Smoking (%)	Follow-up	ISR (%)	Outcome
Shernoff et al. (1994)	100 patients with well-controlled T2DM	NA	178	NA	NA	1 year	92.7	Dental implants can remain functionally stable in patients with well-controlled T2DM.
Balshi and Wolfinger (1999)	34 patients with well-controlled T2DM	62.1	227	NA	5.9	5.9 months	94.3	Dental implants can remain functionally stable in patients with well-controlled T2DM.
Olson et al. (2000)	89 patients with well-controlled T2DM	62.7	178	8.7 years	38	5 years	~88	Dental implants can remain functionally stable in patients with well-controlled T2DM.
Abdulwassie and Dhanrajani (2002)	25 patients with well-controlled T2DM	~47	113	NA	NA	3 years	95.5	Dental implants can remain functionally stable in patients with well-controlled T2DM.
Tawil et al. (2008)	45 with well controlled T2DM 45 Nondiabetics	64.7 59.6	255 244	12.7 years	48.9 40	Up to 12 years	97.2	ISR were comparable among individuals with well-controlled T2DM and controls.
Inbarajan et al. (2012)	5 patients with well controlled T2DM	NA	5	NA	NA	90 days	100	Dental implants can remain functionally stable in patients with well-controlled T2DM.
Malik et al. (2012)	14 patients with well-controlled T2DM	61	28	NA	NA	9 months	100	Dental implants can remain functionally stable in patients with well-controlled T2DM.
Erdogan et al. (2014)	12 with well controlled T2DM 12 Nondiabetics	50	24	NA	NA	1 year	100	Dental implants can remain functionally stable in patients with well-controlled T2DM.
Al Amri et al. (2016)	30 patients with well-controlled T2DM 31 patients with poorly controlled T2DM 30 nondiabetic controls	50.1 50.5 48.5	30 31 30	NA	NA	2 years	100	Dental implants can remain functionally stable in patients with well-controlled T2DM.
Eskow and Oates (2016)	24 with poorly controlled T2DM	59.9	72	14.2	NA	2 years	96.6	Patients with poorly controlled diabetes can undergo dental implant therapy.

T2DM: Type 2 Diabetes mellitus; ISR: Implant success/survival rate; NA: Not available.

Table 9.2 Outcomes of studies assessing the success and survival of dental implants in patients with diabetes.

Authors et al.	Study subjects (n)	Mean age	Study groups	Total implants inserted (n)	Follow-up	Outcome
McCracken et al. (2000)	32 rats	4 months	Poorly controlled diabetes: 20 rats Non-diabetic: 16 rats	32	14 days	Osseointegration was compromised in rats with diabetes as compared to those without diabetes.
Siqueira et al. (2003)	43 rats	3 months	Insulin controlled diabetes: 8 rats Poorly controlled diabetes: 18 rats Non-diabetic: 17 rats	43	Up to 21 days	Osseointegration was compromised in rats with diabetes as compared to those without diabetes. Osseointegration was comparable in well-controlled DM and control rats
Kopman et al. (2005)	32 rats	NA	Diabetic rats on aminoguanidine therapy: 8 rats Diabetic rats on doxycycline therapy: 8 rats Diabetic rats with no treatment: 8 rats Non-diabetic rats with no treatment: 8 rats	32	28 days	Osseointegration was compromised in rats with diabetes as compared to those without diabetes.
Kwon et al. (2005)	32 rats	28 days	Insulin controlled diabetes: 16 rats Poorly controlled diabetes: 16 rats	32	Up to 4 months	Osseointegration was compromised in rats with diabetes as compared to those without diabetes.
McCracken et al. (2006)	152 rats	NA	Insulin controlled diabetes: 32 rats Poorly controlled diabetes: 60 rats Non-diabetic: 60 rats	152	Up to 24 days	Diabetic rats demonstrated significantly more bone associated with implants compared with nondiabetic and insulin groups.
Casap et al. (2008)	140 rats	4 months	Insulin controlled diabetes: 70 rats Poorly controlled diabetes: 70 rats	140	Up to 2 months	No significant difference, in implant osseointegration among diabetic and control rats.
Wang et al. (2011)	20 rats	2 months	Insulin controlled diabetes: 10 rats Poorly controlled diabetes: 10 rats	20	Up to 1.5 months	Osseointegration was compromised in rats with diabetes as compared to those without diabetes. Osseointegration was comparable in well-controlled DM and control rats
Lee et al. (2013)	60 rats	~3 months	Insulin controlled diabetes: 20 rats Poorly controlled diabetes: 20 rats Non-diabetic rats: 20	60	Up to 1.5 months	Hydrophilic titanium domes may present a tendency to promote new bone formation in healthy and diabetic conditions.
de Molon et al. (2013)	80 rats	4 months	2-month controls: 20 rats 4-month controls: 20 rats Insulin-controlled DM: 20 rats Poorly-controlled DM: 20 rats	80	2 months	Osseointegration was comparable in well-controlled DM and control rats as compared to rats with poorly controlled DM.

Characteristics of experimental studies.
In all studies, diabetic rats had fasting blood glucose levels $\geq 200\,mg/dL$.

Al Amri et al., 2016) included, 9 studies (Shernoff et al., 1994; Balshi and Wolfinger, 1999; Olson et al., 2000; Abdulwassie and Dhanrajani, 2002; Tawil et al., 2008; Inbarajan et al., 2012; Malik et al., 2012; Erdogan et al., 2014; Al Amri et al., 2016) were clinical and 9 studies (McCracken et al., 2000; Siqueira et al., 2003; Kopman et al., 2005; Kwon et al., 2005; McCracken et al., 2006; Casap et al., 2008; Wang et al., 2011; Lee et al., 2013; de Molon et al., 2013) were experimental (base on animal models).

In the clinical studies (Shernoff et al., 1994; Balshi and Wolfinger, 1999; Olson et al., 2000; Abdulwassie and Dhanrajani, 2002; Tawil et al., 2008; Inbarajan et al., 2012; Malik et al., 2012; Erdogan et al., 2014; Al Amri et al., 2016) implant survival rates among patients with well-controlled T2DM and nondiabetic individuals were assessed using parameters, such as resonance frequency analysis, periotest, histomorphometry, radiographs, and measurement of clinical parameters of peri-implant inflammation. Six studies (Balshi and Wolfinger, 1999; Olson et al., 2000; Abdulwassie and Dhanrajani, 2002; Tawil et al., 2008; Erdogan et al., 2014; Al Amri et al., 2016) reported mean ages of the study participants, which ranged between ~46 years and 64.7 years. The total numbers of implants inserted ranged between 5 and 255 implants. Duration of DM was reported in studies by Olson et al. (2000) and Tawil et al. (2008), which were 12.7 years and 8.7 years, respectively. In studies by Balshi and Wolfinger (1999), Olson et al. (2000) and Tawil et al. (2008), 48.9%, 5.9%, and 38% of the patients with well-controlled T2DM, respectively, were tobacco smokers. The patients were observed in follow-up periods ranging from 5.9 months and up to 12 years. Results from all clinical studies reported that dental implants can osseointegrate in patients with well-controlled T2DM. In the clinical studies, the overall implant survival rate ranged between ~88% to 100%.

All experimental studies were performed in rats (McCracken et al., 2000; Siqueira et al., 2003; Kopman et al., 2005; Kwon et al., 2005; McCracken et al., 2006; Casap et al., 2008; Wang et al., 2011; Lee et al., 2013; de Molon et al., 2013). The number of study animals used ranged between 20 rats and 140 rats. Seven studies (McCracken et al., 2000; Siqueira et al., 2003; Kwon et al., 2005; Casap et al., 2008; Wang et al., 2011; Lee et al., 2013; de Molon et al., 2013) reported the mean age of animals, which ranged between 14 days to 4 months. In 8 studies (McCracken et al., 2000; Siqueira et al., 2003; Kopman et al., 2005; Kwon et al., 2005; McCracken et al., 2006; Casap et al., 2008; Wang et al., 2011; de Molon et al., 2013), titanium implants were placed in the limbs (tibia or femora), and in one study, dome-shaped titanium discs were placed in standardized-sized defects created in rat calvaria (Lee et al., 2013). The total numbers of implants placed in the animals ranged between 20 implants and 140 implants. In all experimental studies, bone or bone-like tissues present adjacent to the dental implants were quantified using histologic and histomorphometric techniques. The follow-up period ranged from 21 days up to 4 months. Results from five studies (McCracken et al., 2000; Siqueira et al., 2003; Kopman et al., 2005; Kwon et al., 2005; Wang et al., 2011) showed that osseointegration is compromised in rats with diabetes, as compared to those without diabetes. One study reported no significant difference in osseointegration between rats with and without experimentally induced diabetes (Casap et al., 2008). Lee et al. (2013) showed that hydrophilic titanium domes may present a tendency to promote new bone formation in healthy and diabetic conditions. In one study, rats with experimentally induced diabetes demonstrated significantly more bone associated with implants compared with nondiabetic and insulin groups (McCracken et al., 2006). Three studies reported that osseointegration was comparable in well-controlled DM and control rats (Siqueira et al., 2003; Wang et al., 2011; de Molon et al., 2013).

Discussion

The use of dental implants in diabetic patients has been debated upon due to the adverse effects of hyperglycemia on osseointegration (Mombelli and Cionca, 2006; Hasegawa et al., 2008; Messer et al., 2009). Poorly controlled diabetes mellitus may increase the host inflammatory response to oral biofilm, which, in turn, may exacerbate preconditions associated with gingivitis in susceptible individuals (Andriankaja et al., 2009). Moreover, results of Kopman's study using a rat model confirm previous reports that diabetes inhibits osseointegration, as defined by marrow bone-to-implant contact (Kopman et al., 2005). Furthermore, clinical studies have also reported that there is an increased alveolar bone loss in diabetic patients compared to nondiabetic individuals (Javed et al., 2007; Salvi et al., 2008). This may be explained by an increased production of proinflammatory cytokines (such as IL-1β, IL-6, and tumor necrosis factor-alpha [TNF-α]) in the serum and gingival crevicular fluid (GCF) due to the accelerated AGEs-RAGE interactions in diabetic patients (Graves and Cochran, 2003; Graves, 2008). An increased expression of proinflammatory cytokines has also been observed in bone tissues, which supports the idea that bone, by itself, exhibits an inflammatory response in diabetes (Rocha et al., 2001). In general, such mechanisms would probably lead to enhanced formation of osteoclasts and increased bone loss.

A strict glycemic control has been shown to reduce microvascular complications in diabetes (Rocha et al., 2001). It has been reported that maintenance of serum glycemic levels may help to improve the function of osteoblasts, and the progression of periodontal bone loss is markedly reduced in subjects with well-controlled diabetes compared to individuals with poorly controlled diabetes in subjects with diabetes (Taylor et al., 1998). The serum and GCF concentrations of proinflammatory cytokines are also significantly reduced in subjects with well-controlled diabetes compared to individuals with poorly controlled diabetes (Iwamoto et al., 2001; Javed et al., 2014b). Therefore, under optimal glycemic control, diabetic subjects can have a periodontal bone height similar to that of healthy individuals.

Studies on diabetes-induced rat models have shown that insulin therapy is able to up-regulate bone formation around implant (Loe, 1993; Casap et al., 2008). Results from an experimental study showed that osseointegrated dental implants in insulin-controlled diabetic rats maintained bone-to-implant contacts over a 4-month period, whereas in uncontrolled diabetic rats the bone-to-implant contact appears to decrease with time (Kwon et al., 2005). Likewise, clinical studies have also shown that dental implant therapy can be offered to diabetic patients. In a study by Shernoff, Colwell, and Bingham (1994), 178 implants placed in 89 diabetic patients. The results demonstrated a success rate of 92.7% over a year (Shernoff et al., 1994). Moreover, Tawil et al. (2008) reported no significant difference in the implant survival rate between individuals with well-controlled (HbA$_{1c}$ < 7%) diabetes and nondiabetic controls. In this study, the overall implant survival rate for individuals with and without diabetes was similar, that is, 97.2% and 98.8%, respectively (Tawil et al., 2008). However, Dowell et al. found no evidence of compromise in implant success in subjects with poorly controlled diabetes compared to nondiabetic controls (Dowell et al., 2007). Similar results were reported in a two-year follow-up study, which showed a 96.6% survival rate of dental implants placed in patients with poorly controlled diabetes mellitus (Eskow and Oates, 2016).

Immediate functional loading of dental implants is possible, and studies have shown that immediate loading of dental implants (with light forces) does not negatively affect the bone healing-pattern (Romanos et al., 2001; Romanos et al., 2002). Histological and histomorphometric investigations from human retrieved implants after immediate loading have also shown evidence of osseointegration and presence of dense lamellar bone at the interface (Romanos et al., 2005). Studies have shown that a successful osseointegration of immediately loaded dental implants can also be achieved in diabetic patients provided their plasma glucose levels are under normal range (Balshi et al., 2007; Tawil et al., 2008). It has been shown that immediately loaded implants can be successfully osseointegrated in T2DM individuals provided their serum glycemic levels are controlled (Tawil et al. 2008). This may be explained by results from Javed et al. (2007), which showed that periodontal bone loss is markedly reduced in diabetic individuals with optimal glycemic control compared to patients with poorly controlled diabetes.

The influence of age and duration of diabetes on the success of dental implants has also been investigated (Tawil et al., 2008; Koldsland et al., 2009). Tawil et al. (2008) compared the implant survival rates between diabetic and nondiabetic subjects aged ≤ 60 years and > 60 years. The results showed no effect of age on the survival rate of dental implants (Tawil et al., 2008). To evaluate the influence of duration of diabetes on the implant survival rate, Tawil et al. (2008) divided the diabetic patients into four groups (with reference to duration of diabetes), and the results showed no significant differences in implant survival rates between the groups. All diabetic patients participating in this study had well-controlled diabetes, and it may therefore be postulated that under optimal serum glycemic control, the duration of diabetes does not negatively influence the implant survival rate (Tawil et al., 2008).

Although maintenance of serum glycemic levels plays an important role in successful osseointegration, there are other factors that may also assist in enhancing the implant survival rates in diabetic patients. Maintenance of periodontal healthy environment is essential for successful dental implant treatment (Mealey and Oates, 2006). Dental plaque is a major etiological factor in periodontal destruction and studies have reported higher scores of plaque index, BOP and PPD in diabetic patients compared to nondiabetic controls (Javed et al., 2007; Javed et al., 2009). It has been reported that inflammatory periodontal diseases may increase insulin resistance in a way similar to obesity, thereby aggravating glycemic control (Mealey and Oates, 2006). Inflammatory reactions in the peri-implant tissues have been associated with the presence of dental plaque around implants (Maximo et al., 2009). Periodontal therapy has been shown to improve glycemic control in hyperglycemic patients (Javed et al., 2014a). In high-fat-fed diabetic rats, periodontitis accelerated the onset of severe insulin resistance and impaired glucose homeostasis (Watanabe et al., 2008). Therefore, control and treatment of periodontal infections should thus be an important part of the overall management of diabetes mellitus patients and consequently could play an important role for successful implant therapy.

The routine use of antibiotics in oral implantology is widespread; however, there is a controversy over the use of antimicrobial agents in healthy candidates for dental implant therapy (Javed et al., 2013). In diabetic patients undergoing implant surgery, the use of antimicrobial agents reduces the risk of surgical wound infection and improves the implant survival rate. It has been shown that a preoperative antibiotic cover in diabetic patients improves the implant survival rate by 10.5% compared to healthy candidates for implants (improvement with antibiotics was 4.5%) (Morris et al., 2000). In another study, data for 2,973 implants were investigated with reference to success of osseointegration at different stages of implant treatment (Laskin et al., 2000). The results showed that at each stage of treatment, the implant survival rate was notably higher in subjects, who had received preoperative antibiotics (Laskin et al., 2000).

It has been reported that the use of chlorhexidine mouthrinse is effective at reducing the viability of *Porphyromonas gingivalis* infection and peri-implant mucositis (Leyes Borrajo et al., 2002). A twice-daily use of an antiseptic mouthwash has been suggested for the maintenance of dental implants (Ciancio et al., 1995).

Conclusion

In patients with well-controlled T2DM, dental implants can remain functionally stable in a manner similar to nondiabetic individuals. Optimal glycemic control plays a role in the long-term survival of dental implants.

GRADE ACCORDING TO LEVEL OF EVIDENCE: **A**

References

Abdulwassie, H. and Dhanrajani, P. J. 2002. Diabetes mellitus and dental implants: a clinical study. *Implant Dentistry* 11, pp. 83–86.

Al Amri, M. D., Kellesarian, S. V., Al-Kheraif, A. A., Malmstrom, H., Javed, F. and Romanos, G. E. 2016. Effect of oral hygiene maintenance on HbA1c levels and peri-implant parameters around immediately-loaded dental implants placed in type-2 diabetic patients: 2 years follow-up. *Clinical Oral Implants Research* 27, pp. 1439–1443. doi:10.1111/clr.12758.

Andriankaja, O. M., Barros, S. P., Moss, K., Panagakos, F. S., DeVizio, W., Beck, J. and Offenbacher, S. 2009. Levels of serum interleukin (IL)-6 and gingival crevicular fluid of IL-1beta and prostaglandin E(2) among non-smoking subjects with gingivitis and type 2 diabetes. *Journal of Periodontology* 80, pp. 307–316. doi:10.1902/jop.2009.080385.

Balshi, T. J. and Wolfinger, G. J. 1999. Dental implants in the diabetic patient: a retrospective study. *Implant Dentistry* 8, pp. 355–359.

Balshi, S. F., Wolfinger, G. J. and Balshi, T. J. 2007. An examination of immediately loaded dental implant stability in the diabetic patient using resonance frequency analysis (RFA). *Quintessence International* 38, pp. 271–279.

Casap, N., Nimri, S., Ziv, E., Sela, J. and Samuni, Y. 2008. Type 2 diabetes has minimal effect on osseointegration of titanium implants in Psammomys obesus. *Clinical Oral Implants Research* 19, pp. 458–464. doi:10.1111/j.1600-0501.2007.01495.x.

Ciancio, S. G., Lauciello, F., Shibly, O., Vitello, M. and Mather, M. 1995. The effect of an antiseptic mouthrinse on implant maintenance: plaque and peri-implant gingival tissues. *Journal of Periodontology* 66, pp. 962–965. doi:10.1902/jop.1995.66.11.962.

de Molon, R. S., Morais-Camilo, J. A., Verzola, M. H., Faeda, R. S., Pepato, M. T. and Marcantonio, E., Jr. 2013. Impact of diabetes mellitus and metabolic control on bone healing around osseointegrated implants: removal torque and histomorphometric analysis in rats. *Clinical Oral Implants Research* 24, pp. 831–837. doi:10.1111/j.1600-0501.2012.02467.x.

Dowell, S., Oates, T. W. and Robinson, M. 2007. Implant success in people with type 2 diabetes mellitus with varying glycemic control: a pilot study. *The Journal of the American Dental Association* 138, pp. 355–361; quiz 397–358.

Ebersole, J. L., Holt, S. C., Hansard, R. and Novak, M. J. 2008. Microbiologic and immunologic characteristics of periodontal disease in Hispanic Americans with type 2 diabetes. *Journal of Periodontology* 79, pp. 637–646. doi:10.1902/jop.2008.070455.

Erdogan, O., Ucar, Y., Tatli, U., Sert, M., Benlidayi, M. E. and Evlice, B. 2014. A clinical prospective study on alveolar bone augmentation and dental implant success in patients with type 2 diabetes. *Clinical Oral Implants Research.* doi:10.1111/clr.12450.

Eskow, C. C. and Oates, T. W. 2016. Dental implant survival and complication rate over 2 years for individuals with poorly controlled type 2 diabetes mellitus. *Clinical Implant Dentistry and Related Research.* doi:10.1111/cid.12465.

Ferreira, S. D., Silva, G. L., Cortelli, J. R., Costa, J. E. and Costa, F. O. 2006. Prevalence and risk variables for peri-implant disease in Brazilian subjects. *Journal of Clinical Periodontology* 33, pp. 929–935. doi:10.1111/j.1600-051X.2006.01001.x.

Gomez-Moreno, G., Aguilar-Salvatierra, A., Rubio Roldan, J., Guardia, J., Gargallo, J. and Calvo-Guirado, J. L. 2014. Peri-implant evaluation in type 2 diabetes mellitus patients: a 3-year study. *Clinical Oral Implants Research.* doi:10.1111/clr.12391.

Graves, D. 2008. Cytokines that promote periodontal tissue destruction. *Journal of Periodontology* 79, pp. 1585–1591. doi:10.1902/jop.2008.080183.

Graves, D. T. and Cochran, D. 2003. The contribution of interleukin-1 and tumor necrosis factor to periodontal tissue destruction. *Journal of Periodontology* 74, pp. 391–401. doi:10.1902/jop.2003.74.3.391.

Hasegawa, H., Ozawa, S., Hashimoto, K., Takeichi, T. and Ogawa, T. 2008. Type 2 diabetes impairs implant osseointegration capacity in rats. *International Journal of Oral and Maxillofacial Implants* 23, pp. 237–246.

Holla, L. I., Kankova, K., Fassmann, A., Buckova, D., Halabala, T., Znojil, V. and Vanek, J. 2001. Distribution of the receptor for advanced glycation end products gene polymorphisms in patients with chronic periodontitis: a preliminary study. *Journal of Periodontology* 72, pp. 1742–1746. doi:10.1902/jop.2001.72.12.1742.

Inbarajan, A., Veeravalli, P. T., Vaidyanathan, A. K. and Grover, M. 2012. Short-term evaluation of dental implants in a diabetic population: an in vivo study. *Journal of Advanced Prosthodontics* 4, pp. 134–138. doi:10.4047/jap.2012.4.3.134.

Iwamoto, Y., Nishimura, F., Nakagawa, M., Sugimoto, H., Shikata, K., Makino, H., Fukuda, T., Tsuji, T., Iwamoto, M. and Murayama, Y. 2001. The effect of antimicrobial periodontal treatment on circulating tumor necrosis factor-alpha and glycated hemoglobin level in patients with type 2 diabetes. *Journal of Periodontology* 72, pp. 774–778. doi:10.1902/jop.2001.72.6.774.

Javed, F., Ahmed, H. B., Mehmood, A., Bain, C. and Romanos, G. E. 2014a. Effect of nonsurgical periodontal therapy (with or without oral doxycycline delivery) on glycemic status and clinical periodontal parameters in patients with prediabetes: a short-term longitudinal randomized case-control study. *Clinical Oral Investing.* doi:10.1007/s00784-014-1185-6.

Javed, F., Al-Daghri, N. M., Wang, H. L., Wang, C. Y. and Al-Hezaimi, K. 2014b. Short-term effects of non-surgical periodontal treatment on the gingival crevicular fluid cytokine profiles in sites with induced periodontal defects: a study on dogs with and without streptozotocin-induced diabetes. *Journal of Periodontology,* pp. 1–11. doi:10.1902/jop.2014.140150.

Javed, F., Alghamdi, A. S., Ahmed, A., Mikami, T., Ahmed, H. B. and Tenenbaum, H. C. 2013. Clinical efficacy of antibiotics in the treatment of peri-implantitis. *International Dental Journal* 63, pp. 169–176. doi:10.1111/idj.12034.

Javed, F., Klingspor, L., Sundin, U., Altamash, M., Klinge, B. and Engstrom, P. E. 2009. Periodontal conditions, oral Candida albicans and salivary proteins in type 2 diabetic subjects with emphasis on gender. *BMC Oral Health* 9, pp. 12. doi:10.1186/1472-6831-9-12.

Javed, F., Nasstrom, K., Benchimol, D., Altamash, M., Klinge, B. and Engstrom, P. E. 2007. Comparison of periodontal and socioeconomic status between subjects with type 2 diabetes mellitus and non-diabetic controls. *Journal of Periodontology* 78, pp. 2112–2119. doi:10.1902/jop.2007.070186.

Javed, F. and Romanos, G. E. 2009. Impact of diabetes mellitus and glycemic control on the osseointegration of dental implants: a systematic literature review. *Journal of Periodontology* 80, pp. 1719–1730. doi:10.1902/jop.2009.090283.

Koldsland, O. C., Scheie, A. A. and Aass, A. M. 2009. Prevalence of implant loss and the influence of associated factors. *Journal of Periodontology* 80, pp. 1069–1075. doi:10.1902/jop.2009.080594.

Kopman, J. A., Kim, D. M., Rahman, S. S., Arandia, J. A., Karimbux, N. Y. and Fiorellini, J. P. 2005. Modulating the effects of diabetes on osseointegration with aminoguanidine and doxycycline. *Journal of Periodontology* 76, pp. 614–620. doi:10.1902/jop.2005.76.4.614.

Kwon, P. T., Rahman, S. S., Kim, D. M., Kopman, J. A., Karimbux, N. Y. and Fiorellini, J. P. 2005. Maintenance of osseointegration utilizing insulin therapy in a diabetic rat model. *Journal of Periodontology* 76, pp. 621–626. doi:10.1902/jop.2005.76.4.621.

Laskin, D. M., Dent, C. D., Morris, H. F., Ochi, S. and Olson, J. W. 2000. The influence of preoperative antibiotics on success of endosseous implants at 36 months. *Annals of Periodontology* 5, pp. 166–174. doi:10.1902/annals.2000.5.1.166.

Lee, S. B., Retzepi, M., Petrie, A., Hakimi, A. R., Schwarz, F. and Donos, N. 2013. The effect of diabetes on bone formation following application of the GBR principle with the use of titanium domes. *Clinical Oral Implants Research* 24, pp. 28–35. doi:10.1111/j.1600-0501.2012.02448.x.

Leyes Borrajo, J. L., Garcia, V. L., Lopez, C. G., Rodriguez-Nunez, I., Garcia, F. M. and Gallas, T. M. 2002. Efficacy of chlorhexidine mouthrinses with and without alcohol: a clinical study. *Journal of Periodontology* 73, pp. 317–321. doi:10.1902/jop.2002.73.3.317.

Loe, H. 1993. Periodontal disease. The sixth complication of diabetes mellitus. *Diabetes Care* 16, pp. 329–334.

Mager, D. R., Iniguez, I. R., Gilmour, S. and Yap, J. 2013. The effect of a low fructose and low glycemic index/load (fragile) dietary intervention on indices of liver function, cardiometabolic risk factors, and body composition in children and adolescents with nonalcoholic fatty liver disease (NAFLD). *Journal of Parenteral and Enteral Nutrition* doi:10.1177/0148607113501201.

Malik, A., Shaari, R., Rahman, S. A. and Aljuboori, M. J. 2012. Influence of platelet-rich plasma on dental implants. Osseointegration in well-controlled diabetic patients. *Dental Implantolology Update* 23, pp. 89–96.

Maximo, M. B., de Mendonca, A. C., Renata Santos, V., Figueiredo, L. C., Feres, M. and Duarte, P. M. 2009. Short-term clinical and microbiological evaluations of peri-implant diseases before and after mechanical anti-infective therapies. *Clinical Oral Implants Research* 20, pp. 99–108. doi:10.1111/j.1600-0501.2008.01618.x.

McCracken, M., Lemons, J. E., Rahemtulla, F., Prince, C. W. and Feldman, D. 2000. Bone response to titanium alloy implants placed in diabetic rats. *International Journal of Oral and Maxillofacial Implants* 15, pp. 345–354.

McCracken, M. S., Aponte-Wesson, R., Chavali, R. and Lemons, J. E. 2006. Bone associated with implants in diabetic and insulin-treated rats. *Clinical Oral Implants Research* 17, pp. 495–500. doi:10.1111/j.1600-0501.2006.01266.x.

Mealey, B. L. and Oates, T. W. 2006. Diabetes mellitus and periodontal diseases. *Journal of Periodontology* 77, pp. 1289–1303. doi:10.1902/jop.2006.050459.

Messer, R. L., Tackas, G., Mickalonis, J., Brown, Y., Lewis, J. B. and Wataha, J. C. 2009. Corrosion of machined titanium dental implants under inflammatory conditions. *Journal of Biomedical Materials Research Part B: Applied Biomaterials* 88, pp. 474–481. doi:10.1002/jbm.b.31162.

Mombelli, A. and Cionca, N. 2006. Systemic diseases affecting osseointegration therapy. *Clinical Oral Implants Research* 17 Suppl 2, pp. 97–103. doi:10.1111/j.1600-0501.2006.01354.x.

Morris, H. F., Ochi, S. and Winkler, S. 2000. Implant survival in patients with type 2 diabetes: placement to 36 months. *Annals of Periodontology* 5, pp. 157–165. doi:10.1902/annals.2000.5.1.157.

Murillo, J., Wang, Y., Xu, X., Klebe, R. J., Chen, Z., Zardeneta, G., Pal, S., Mikhailova, M. and Steffensen, B. 2008. Advanced glycation of type I collagen and fibronectin modifies periodontal cell behavior. *Journal of Periodontology* 79, pp. 2190–2199. doi:10.1902/jop.2008.080210.

Oates, T. W., Dowell, S., Robinson, M. and McMahan, C. A. 2009. Glycemic control and implant stabilization in type 2 diabetes mellitus. *Journal of Dental Research* 88, pp. 367–371. doi:10.1177/0022034509334203.

Olson, J. W., Shernoff, A. F., Tarlow, J. L., Colwell, J. A., Scheetz, J. P. and Bingham, S. F. 2000. Dental endosseous implant assessments in a type 2 diabetic population: a prospective study. *International Journal of Oral and Maxillofacial Implants* 15, pp. 811–818.

Rocha, M., Nava, L. E., Vazquez de la Torre, C., Sanchez-Marin, F., Garay-Sevilla, M. E. and Malacara, J. M. 2001. Clinical and radiological improvement of periodontal disease in patients with type 2 diabetes mellitus treated with alendronate: a randomized, placebo-controlled trial. *Journal of Periodontology* 72, pp. 204–209. doi:10.1902/jop.2001.72.2.204.

Romanos, G., Toh, C. G., Siar, C. H., Swaminathan, D., Ong, A. H., Donath, K., Yaacob, H. and Nentwig, G. H. 2001. Peri-implant bone reactions to immediately loaded implants. *An experimental study in monkeys. Journal of Periodontology* 72, pp. 506–511. doi:10.1902/jop.2001.72.4.506.

Romanos, G. E., Toh, C. G., Siar, C. H. and Swaminathan, D. 2002. Histologic and histomorphometric evaluation of peri-implant bone subjected to immediate loading: an experimental study with Macaca fascicularis. *International Journal of Oral and Maxillofacial Implants* 17, pp. 44–51.

Romanos, G.E., Testori, T., Degidi, M. and Piattelli, A. 2005. Histologic and histomorphometric findings from retrieved, immediately occlusally loaded implants in humans. *Journal of Periodontology* 76, pp. 1823–1832.

Salvi, G. E., Carollo-Bittel, B. and Lang, N. P. 2008. Effects of diabetes mellitus on periodontal and peri-implant conditions: update on associations and risks. *Journal of Clinical Periodontology* 35, pp. 398–409. doi:10.1111/j.1600-051X.2008.01282.x.

Shernoff, A. F., Colwell, J. A. and Bingham, S. F. 1994. Implants for type II diabetic patients: interim report. VA Implants in Diabetes Study Group. *Implant Dentistry* 3, pp. 183–185.

Siqueira, J. T., Cavalher-Machado, S. C., Arana-Chavez, V. E. and Sannomiya, P. 2003. Bone formation around titanium implants in the rat tibia: role of insulin. *Implant Dentistry* 12, pp. 242–251.

Soory, M. 2002. Hormone mediation of immune responses in the progression of diabetes, rheumatoid arthritis and periodontal diseases. *Current Drug Targets – Immune Endocrine and Metabolic Disorders* 2, pp. 13–25.

Tawil, G., Younan, R., Azar, P. and Sleilati, G. 2008. Conventional and advanced implant treatment in the type II diabetic patient: surgical protocol and long-term clinical results. *International Journal of Oral and Maxillofacial Implants* 23, pp. 744–752.

Taylor, G. W., Burt, B. A., Becker, M. P., Genco, R. J. and Shlossman, M. 1998. Glycemic control and alveolar bone loss progression in type 2 diabetes. *Annals of Periodontology* 3, pp. 30–39. doi:10.1902/annals.1998.3.1.30.

Wang, B., Song, Y., Wang, F., Li, D., Zhang, H., Ma, A. and Huang, N. 2011. Effects of local infiltration of insulin around titanium implants in diabetic rats. *British Journal of Oral and Maxillofacial Surgery* 49, pp. 225–229. doi:10.1016/j.bjoms.2010.03.006.

Watanabe, K., Petro, B. J., Shlimon, A. E. and Unterman, T. G. 2008. Effect of periodontitis on insulin resistance and the onset of type 2 diabetes mellitus in Zucker diabetic fatty rats. *Journal of Periodontology* 79, pp. 1208–1216. doi:10.1902/jop.2008.070605.

10

Impact of Oral Cancer Therapy on the Survival of Dental Implants

Introduction

Surgical excision of oral malignancies is often followed by either radiotherapy or chemotherapy or both. The overall impression regarding the success of dental implants in patients having undergone oral cancer therapy remains unclear. Irradiated sites are more susceptible to tissue necrosis and consequent loss of implants compared to nonirradiated sites (Granstrom et al., 1992). In a study on 131 dental implants placed in 27 patients having undergone radiotherapy, a significantly lower implant survival rate (ISR) was noticed (Cao and Weischer, 2003). However, some studies have reported that DI installed in patients having undergone oral cancer therapy, can osseointegrate and remain functionally stable over long durations (Schoen et al., 2007; Korfage et al., 2010). The aim of this chapter is to assess the ISR after oral cancer therapy.

Overview of Studies

Table 10.1 summarizes the studies in which ISR was assessed in patients having undergone oral cancer therapy. From the literature reviewed, it seems that the survival and functional stability of dental implants is higher in the mandible as compared to the maxilla; however, it should be noted that in all the studies, implants were inserted exclusively in the mandible; with the exception of the studies by Niimi et al. (1998) and Visch et al. (2002), in which implants were placed in the mandible as well as the maxilla. Results by Visch et al. (2002) showed the ISR to be slightly higher in the posterior – as compared to the anterior maxilla; however, the difference was not statistically significant. In the Niimi study (1998), the number of implants inserted in the maxilla was too low to depict any definite conclusions; yet, it may be speculated that poor bone quality of the maxilla (which was not assessed in the Niimi study [1998]) could be associated with the poor ISR.

Due to a scarcity of indexed literature on this regard, it is difficult to determine the role of jaw location on the survival of dental implants in patients having undergone oral cancer therapy. Moreover, osteoradionecrosis is usually observed several years after radiotherapy and is associated with local trauma within the hypovascular–hypocellular hypoxic tissues (which occurs as a result of radiation-induced endarteritis) (Marx, 1983; Marx and Johnson, 1987). Thus, the interval between the end of oral cancer therapy and installation of implants may contribute to the success or failure of osseointegration.

Evidence-based Implant Dentistry and Systemic Conditions, First Edition.
Fawad Javed and Georgios E. Romanos.
© 2018 John Wiley & Sons, Inc. Published 2018 by John Wiley & Sons, Inc.

Table 10.1 Outcomes of studies assessing the success and survival of dental implants in patients with oral cancer.

Author/s et al. Year	Subject/s (mean age/ range in years)	Mean radiation dosage in Gy* (range)	Interval†	Dental implants inserted (n)	Follow-up	Implant success rate	Conclusion
Niimi et al. 1998	22 patients from each center (NA‡/ NA‡)	NA‡ (<25 to >66)	NA‡	228	Up to 2 years	88.9% (Japan center) 86% (US center)	Dental implants can osseointegrate and remain functionally stable in patients having undergone therapy for oral malignancy.
Weischer and Mohr 1999	40 (55/43–75)	50 (36–72)	13 months	175	10 years	91%	Irradiated patients should be restored with exclusively implant-supported prostheses, without any mucosal contact.
Kovács 2000	45 (53.5 in males/ range: NA‡ 49.1 in females/ range: NA‡)	—	At least 6 months	162	6 years	97.6%	Dental implants can osseointegrate and remain functionally stable in patients having undergone surgery and chemotherapy.
Kovács 2001	30 (55/ NA‡)	—	10.5 months	106	10 years	99.1%	Chemotherapy did not have detrimental effects on the survival and success of dental implants in oral cancer patients.
Visch et al. 2002	130 (62/34–87)	NA‡ (0 to >72)	At least 6 months	446	14 years	78%	Implant survival is significantly influenced by location, extent of surgery and by the irradiation dose at the implant site.
Cao and Weischer 2003	27 (NA‡/45–79)	NA‡ (36–76)	6 months	131	At least 2 years	88%	DI# supported prosthesis have significantly lower survival rates in irradiated patients compared to nonirradiated patients.
Schoen et al. 2007	26 (60.1/47–77)	61.4 (46–116)	At least 1 year	103	3 years	93.9%	Dental implants can osseointegrate and remain functionally stable in patients having undergone therapy for OSCC§.
Korfage et al. 2010	50 (61.5/41–81)	>40 (12–70)	—	195	5 years	89.4%	DI# can osseointegrate and remain functionally stable in oral cancer patients having undergone surgery and radiotherapy.

*Gray (Unit: Joules/kilogram)
†Interval between conclusion of radiotherapy and dental implant installation
‡Not available
#DI: dental implant
§Oral squamous cell carcinoma

Various studies (Marx and Johnson, 1987; Werkmeister et al., 1999; Kovács, 2000; Kovács, 2001; Visch et al., 2002) have investigated the required time interval between radiotherapy and implant installation that may influence osseointegration; however, the results remain debatable. Marx and Johnson (1987) reported that the risk of oral complications (particularly osteoradionecrosis) and the probability of implant failure is higher in cases where dental implants are inserted between one and six months following radiotherapy. Similar results were reported by another study (Cao and Weischer, 2003) where dental implants, installed six months following irradiation, demonstrated significantly lower ISR. However, the Visch et al. (2002) study reported no significant differences in the survival of dental implants inserted less than 12 months (76%) or at least one year (81%) after radiotherapy. In the Werkmeister study, osseointegration was reported to be negatively influenced in two years following end-of-radiation therapy, and the ISR in nonirradiated bone was also reported to be low (approximately 68%) (Werkmeister et al., 1999). It is challenging to reach a definitive conclusion regarding the influence of interval on the survival of dental implants in patients having undergone chemotherapy. Likewise, there is no consistency in the follow-up durations after installation of dental implants in these patients. Further prospective studies with long-term follow-up are needed to elucidate the effects of radiotherapy on the survival and stability of dental implants. From the two studies (Kovács, 2000; 2001) in which patients had undergone chemotherapy, it seems that dental implants can successfully osseointegrate and remain functionally stable when inserted at least six months after therapy. Also, in these studies, the follow-up examinations were performed after at least five years of implant placement. Therefore, it is suggested that dental implants may remain functionally stable after chemotherapy. Since only a limited number of studies (Kovács, 2000; 2001) have investigated the impact of chemotherapy on stability and function of dental implants in oral cancer patients, further studies are warranted in this regard.

Conclusion
Dental implants can osseointegrate and remain functionally stable in patients having undergone oral cancer therapy; however, such patients should be required to give prior consent to implants with full disclosure regarding possible complications associated with implant treatment following irradiation. GRADE ACCORDING TO LEVEL OF EVIDENCE: **B**

References

Cao, Y. and Weischer, T. 2003. Comparison of maxillary implant-supported prosthesis in irradiated and non-irradiated patients. *Journal of Huazhong University of Science and Technologu Medical Sciences* 23, 209–212.

Granstrom, G., Jacobsson, M. and Tjellstrom, A. 1992. Titanium implants in irradiated tissue: benefits from hyperbaric oxygen. *International Journal of Oral and Maxillofacial Implants* 7, 15–25.

Korfage, A., Schoen, P. J., Raghoebar, G. M., Roodenburg, J. L., Vissink, A. and Reintsema, H. 2010. Benefits of dental implants installed during ablative tumour surgery in oral cancer patients: a prospective 5-year clinical trial. *Clinical Oral Implants Research* 21, 971–979. doi:10.1111/j.1600-0501.2010.01930.x.

Kovács, A. F. 2000. The fate of osseointegrated implants in patients following oral cancer surgery and mandibular reconstruction. *Head Neck* 22, 111–119.

Kovács, A. F. 2001. Influence of chemotherapy on endosteal implant survival and success in oral cancer patients. *International Journal of Oral and Maxillofacial Surgery* 30, 144–147. doi:10.1054/ijom.2000.0023.

Marx, R. E. 1983. Osteoradionecrosis: a new concept of its pathophysiology. *Journal of Oral Maxillofacial Surgery* 41, 283–288.

Marx, R. E. and Johnson, R. P. 1987. Studies in the radiobiology of osteoradionecrosis and their clinical significance. *Oral Surgery, Oral Medicine, and Oral Pathology* 64, 379–390.

Niimi, A., Ueda, M., Keller, E. E. and Worthington, P. 1998. Experience with osseointegrated implants placed in irradiated tissues in Japan and the United States. *Int J Oral Maxillofac Implants* 13, 407–411.

Schoen, P. J., Raghoebar, G. M., Bouma, J., Reintsema, H., Vissink, A., Sterk, W. and Roodenburg, J. L. 2007. Rehabilitation of oral function in head and neck cancer patients after radiotherapy with implant-retained dentures: effects of hyperbaric oxygen therapy. *Oral Oncology* 43, 379–388. doi:10.1016/j.oraloncology.2006.04.009.

Visch, L. L., van Waas, M. A., Schmitz, P. I. and Levendag, P. C. 2002. A clinical evaluation of implants in irradiated oral cancer patients. *Journal of Dental Research* 81, 856–859. doi:10.1177/154405910208101212.

Werkmeister, R., Szulczewski, D., Walteros-Benz, P. and Joos, U. 1999. Rehabilitation with dental implants of oral cancer patients. *Journal of Cranio-Maxillo-Facial Surgery* 27, 38–41.

11

Oral Cancer Arising around Dental Implants

Introduction

Studies have shown that dental implants can exhibit high survival rates in patients having undergone oral cancer treatment (Javed et al., 2010). However, some studies have reported the occurrence of oral squamous cell carcinoma (OSCC) after dental implant therapy (Czerninski et al., 2006; Eguia del Valle et al., 2008; Gallego et al., 2008; Kwok et al., 2008; Gallego et al., 2009; Gulati et al., 2009; De Ceulaer et al., 2010; Meijer et al., 2010). Oral cancer (precisely, OSCC) around dental implants may present as a red, hyperplastic, and or ulcerated oral mucosa with alveolar bone loss and hence may be misdiagnosed as peri-implantitis (Eguia et al., 2008). Under such circumstances, a detailed clinical and radiological evaluation accompanied by a biopsy and histopathologic assessment may be performed to elucidate any diagnostic doubt. Gallego et al. (2008) presented a case-report of an 81-year-old female who had received dental implant therapy. Nearly three years after implant therapy the patient developed an exophytic mass around dental implants, which upon biopsy was diagnosed as OSCC (Gallego et al., 2008). Similarly, Czerninski et al. (2006) presented a case-series of individuals in whom dental implants were placed as a replacement for missing teeth. The individuals included in these studies developed nonhealing ulcers around dental implants a few years after implant therapy. The ulcerated lesions were subjected to histological assessment and the results revealed the presence of OSCC around dental implants (Czerninski et al., 2006). Studies that have shown the occurrence of OSCC around dental implants are summarized in Table 11.1.

Most of the patients that develop OSCC around dental implants have a previous history of some form of cancer (Gallego et al., 2008; Kwok et al., 2008; Gulati et al., 2009). In the Dib study, the patient presented with OSCC seven months after dental implant therapy; however, the patient had a previous history of breast cancer (Dib et al., 2007). Although metastasis to the oral cavity and the jaws are uncommon (estimated to comprise about 1% of newly diagnosed oral malignancies) (Scipio et al., 2001; Ogutcen-Toller et al., 2002); the fact that cellular metastasis of systemic malignancies into the oral cavity cannot be disregarded. Trauma has been reported to facilitate the growth of blood-borne tumors (Tseng et al., 1998). This possibility stems from the entrapment of tumor cells during clot formation in fresh wounds and to the fact that malignant cells grow more rapidly in areas of high cellular proliferation, such as regenerating tissue, mediated by host-generated growth factors. This may be an explanation for the metastasis of malignant cells from different locations into the oral cavity. Though malignant cells are known for their ability to invade different anatomical structures of the body, the role

Evidence-based Implant Dentistry and Systemic Conditions, First Edition.
Fawad Javed and Georgios E. Romanos.
© 2018 John Wiley & Sons, Inc. Published 2018 by John Wiley & Sons, Inc.

Table 11.1 Outcomes of studies assessing the success and survival of dental implants in patients with oral cancer.

Authors et al. (Year)	Study design	Study individual/s	Mean age and (range) in years	Number of implants inserted	Number of cases/ implants associated with OSSC	Outcome
Dib et al. (2007)	Case-report	1 female	67-year-old	8	4 implants	Approximately seven months after implant treatment, inflammatory lesions were seen around the maxillary and mandibular DI. Biopsy confirmed it to be metastatic carcinoma from the breast to jaws.
Eguia et al. (2008)	Case-report	1 male	76-year-old	2	1 implant	The patient presented with a white exophytic lesion (6 mm in diameter), with superficial ulceration. Incisional biopsy showed the presence of a well-differentiated OSCC.
Kwok et al. (2008)	Case-series	1 male 1 male 1 female	62-year-old 71-year-old 67-year-old	14 NA 2	—	Three-months after implant treatment, a non-healing ulcer was seen in the peri-implant tissue on the lingual aspect of the mandibular right premolar region. On biopsy, it was diagnosed as OSCC.
					1 implant	Six years after implant treatment, the patient developed inflammatory changes around one implant. Biopsy revealed the presence of a well-differentiated OSCC.
					1 implant	One year after implant treatment, the patient developed an area of papillary hyperplasia opn the lower lip. Biopsy revealed the presence of OSCC.
Gallego et al. (2009)	Case-report	1 female	70-year-old	3	—	After 12-months of follow-up, no evidence of local or cervical recurrence was observed.
Gulati et al. (2009)	Case-report	1 female	62-year-old	5	2 implants	After extensive oral surgery, the patient suffered from multiple episodes of peri-implantitis and later developed OSCC.
De Ceulaer et al. (2010)	Retrospective	21 (9 males:12 females)	65.8 (27–77)	56	3 patients	Three patients developed local OSCC recurrence around one of the implants. No recurrence of OSCC was observed in the group implanted in second stage surgery.
Meijer et al. (2010)	Case-report	1 female	65-year-old	2	2 implants	Four years after implant therapy, OSCC was observed in the floor of the mouth between the two implants. It extended to the attached keratinized peri-implant mucosa of both implants.

of confounding factors that may also participate in inducing or exacerbating OSSC in dental implant patients cannot be disregarded.

Peri-implantitis is a chronic inflammatory condition, which, if left untreated, may cause progressive loss of supporting bone in the tissues surrounding a functioning implant. In some instances, OSCC may manifest clinical and radiological features (such as mucosal hyperplasia, mucosal ulcerations, and alveolar bone loss) similar to peri-implantitis (Jane-Salas et al., 2012). The gingival attachment around dental implants is an area that experiences constant inflammation, which may, in turn, affect mucosal stability. This inflammation may play an important role in the development of cancer due to the action of cytokine mediators, including interleukin-1, interleukin-6, and tumor necrosis factor (Jane-Salas et al., 2012). A biopsy and histopathological assessment is particularly essential when mucosal inflammation and alveolar bone loss rapidly occur around dental implants without any response to therapy. This may assist in clarifying any diagnostic doubts.

A limitation of this chapter is that the study search yielded only case-reports or case-series; however, further prospective studies are warranted to comprehend the development of OSCC around osseointegrated dental implants.

Conclusion
OSCC is more likely to arise around osseointegrated DI in patients with a previous history of cancer. The role of other factors including tobacco and alcohol usage cannot be disregarded.
GRADE ACCORDING TO LEVEL OF EVIDENCE: **C**

References

Czerninski, R., Kaplan, I., Almoznino, G., Maly, A. and Regev, E. 2006. Oral squamous cell carcinoma around dental implants. *Quintessence International (Berlin, Germany : 1985)* 37: pp. 707–711.

De Ceulaer, J., Magremanne, M., van Veen, A. and Scheerlinck, J. 2010. Squamous cell carcinoma recurrence around dental implants. *Journal of Oral and Maxillofacial Surgery: official journal of the American Association of Oral and Maxillofacial Surgeons* 68: pp. 2507–2512.

Dib, L. L., Soares, A. L., Sandoval, R. L. and Nannmark, U. 2007. Breast metastasis around dental implants: A case report. *Clinical Implant Dentistry and Related Research* 9: pp. 112–115.

Eguia del Valle, A., Martinez-Conde Llamosas, R., Lopez Vicente, J., Uribarri Etxebarria, A. and Aguirre Urizar, J. M. 2008. Primary oral squamous cell carcinoma arising around dental osseointegrated implants mimicking peri-implantitis. *Medicina oral, patologia oral y cirugia bucal* 13: pp. E489–491.

Gallego, L., Junquera, L., Baladron, J. and Villarreal, P. 2008. Oral squamous cell carcinoma associated with symphyseal dental implants: An unusual case report. *Journal of the American Dental Association (1939)* 139: pp. 1061–1065.

Gallego, L., Junquera, L. and Llorente, S. 2009. Oral carcinoma associated with implant-supported overdenture trauma: A case report. *Dental traumatology: official publication of International Association for Dental Traumatology* 25: pp. e3–4.

Gulati, A., Puthussery, F. J., Downie, I. P. and Flood, T. R. 2009. Squamous cell carcinoma presenting as peri-implantitis: A case report. *Annals of the Royal College of Surgeons of England* 91: pp. W8–10.

Jane-Salas, E., Lopez-Lopez, J., Rosello-Llabres, X., Rodriguez-Argueta, O. F. and Chimenos-Kustner, E. 2012. Relationship between oral cancer and implants: Clinical cases and systematic literature review. *Medicina oral, patologia oral y cirugia bucal* 17: pp. e23–28.

Javed, F., Al-Hezaimi, K., Al-Rasheed, A., Almas, K. and Romanos, G. E. 2010. Implant survival rate after oral cancer therapy: A review. *Oral Oncology* 46: pp. 854–859.

Kwok, J., Eyeson, J., Thompson, I. and McGurk, M. 2008. Dental implants and squamous cell carcinoma in the at risk patient—report of three cases. *British Dental Journal* 205: pp. 543–545.

Meijer, G. J., Dieleman, F. J., Berge, S. J. and Merkx, M. A. 2010. Removal of an oral squamous cell carcinoma including parts of osseointegrated implants in the marginal mandibulectomy. *A case report. Journal of Oral and Maxillofacial Surgery* 14: pp. 253–256.

Ogutcen-Toller, M., Metin, M. and Yildiz, L. 2002. Metastatic breast carcinoma mimicking periodontal disease on radiographs. *Journal of Clinical Periodontology* 29: 269–271.

Scipio, J. E., Murti, P. R., Al-Bayaty, H. F., Matthews, R. and Scully, C. 2001. Metastasis of breast carcinoma to mandibular gingiva. *Oral Oncology* 37: pp. 393–396.

Tseng, L. N., Berends, F. J., Wittich, P., Bouvy, N. D., Marquet, R. L., Kazemier, G. and Bonjer, H. J. 1998. Port-site metastases. Impact of local tissue trauma and gas leakage. *Surgical Endoscopy* 12: pp. 1377–1380.

12

Dental Implants in Patients with Periodontitis

Introduction

Periodontitis encompasses various pathological conditions that jeopardize the periodontium and is usually present in a chronic form (Boutin et al., 2017; Dr et al., 2017); whereas peri-implantitis is defined as the presence of progressive inflammation of the peri-implant mucosa leading to simultaneous loss of supporting bone (Romanos et al., 2015). Mombelli and associates described peri-implantitis as a site-specific infection, which exhibits features similar to those of chronic periodontitis (CP) (Mombelli et al., 1987). Studies have shown that pathogenic microbes associated with CP and peri-implantitis are similar and are mainly composed of Gram-negative anaerobes (Paster et al., 2001; Dingsdag et al., 2016). The classical risk factors of peri-implant diseases (such as peri-implant mucositis and peri-implantitis) include smoking, poor oral hygiene, and an immunocompromised state. However, another factor that has been associated with a higher incidence of biological complications and compromised implant survival rate is a history of CP (Heitz-Mayfield, 2008; Klinge and Meyle, 2012). Nevertheless, the progression of infection around implants and natural teeth is divergent as biological differences exist between natural teeth and dental implants. Moreover, tissues around implants are more prone to plaque-associated infections that spread into the alveolar bone (Lindhe et al., 1992) (see Figures 12.1 to 12.7).

Dental Implants in Patients with a History of Chronic Periodontitis

Studies assessing the outcome of dental implant therapy among patients with a history of CP have shown varying results (Watson et al., 1999; Karoussis et al., 2003; Roos-Jansaker et al., 2006; Ong et al., 2008; Greenstein et al., 2010; Safii et al., 2010; Roccuzzo et al., 2014). Some studies have shown that patients with a history of CP are more susceptible to peri-implant complications, such as increased probing depth and crestal bone loss [CBL] and implant failure, as compared to individuals without a history of CP (Evian et al., 2004; Roos-Jansaker et al., 2006a; Roos-Jansaker et al., 2006b; De Boever et al., 2009; Safii et al., 2010); whereas, others showed no difference in the outcome of dental implant therapy among patients with and without CP (Watson et al., 1999). These results are summarized in Table 12.1.

Dental Implants in Patients with Treated Generalized Aggressive Periodontitis

Although CP is the most common form of periodontal disease, aggressive periodontitis (AgP) is less frequent (Monje et al., 2014). However, the presence of potential risks, such as AgP, may also influence implant success/survival (Albandar and Tinoco, 2002).

Evidence-based Implant Dentistry and Systemic Conditions, First Edition.
Fawad Javed and Georgios E. Romanos.
© 2018 John Wiley & Sons, Inc. Published 2018 by John Wiley & Sons, Inc.

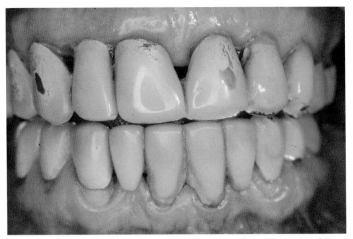

Figure 12.1 Clinical situation presenting the periodontal condition before treatment. (*Source*: Romanos, 2012. Reproduced with permission of Quintessence).

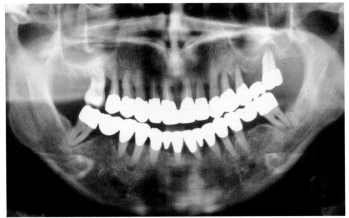

Figure 12.2 Radiographical evaluation of the hopeless dentition. (*Source*: Romanos, 2012. Reproduced with permission of Quintessence).

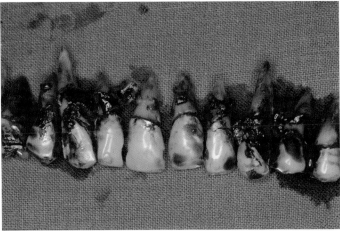

Figure 12.3 Extracted hopeless teeth due to advanced periodontitis. (*Source*: Romanos, 2012. Reproduced with permission of Quintessence).

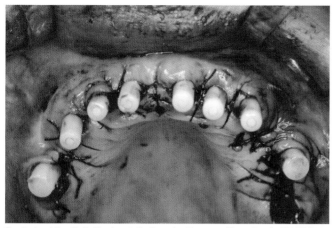

Figure 12.4 Maxillary implants with abutments immediately before fabrication of a chair-side provisionalization.

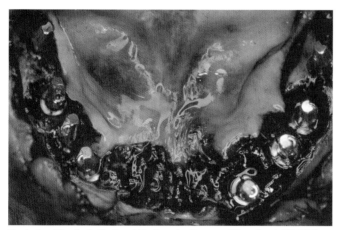

Figure 12.5 Mandibular implants at the day of placement prepared for immediate loading. (*Source*: Romanos, 2012. Reproduced with permission of Quintessence).

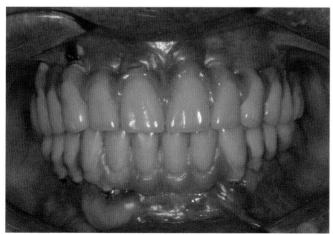

Figure 12.6 Clinical situation 15 years after implant placement with immediate loading.

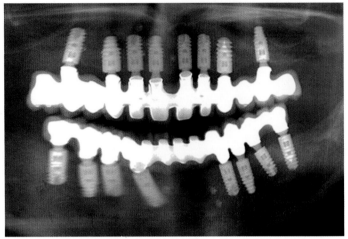

Surgical and Prosthetic Treatment: Dr. Georgios Romanos (Stony Brook, NY, USA)
Dental technician: M. Funk (Bad Vilbel, Germany)

Figure 12.7 Radiographic condition 15 years after treatment presenting the crestal bone stability.

A systematic review and meta-analysis concluded that implant placement in patients with a history of generalized AgP (GAgP) might be considered a viable option to restore oral function with survival outcomes comparable to those found in both patients with CP and healthy controls (Monje et al., 2014). Nevertheless, the authors also concluded that the risk ratio for failure in patients with generalized AgP is significantly higher when compared with healthy controls (Monje et al., 2014). Results from a 10-year follow-up study showed that dental implants can osseointegrate and remain functionally stable in partially edentulous subjects treated for GAgP (Mengel et al., 2007). However, the bone and attachment loss at the implants is higher than in individuals with a healthy periodontal status (Mengel et al., 2007). Similar results were reported in other studies of up to five years follow-up (Mengel et al., 2001; Mengel and Flores-de-Jacoby, 2005). However, results from a prospective study on 35 patients treated for GAgP and 18 periodontally healthy controls showed that patients with treated GAgP are more susceptible to peri-implant diseases (peri-implant mucositis and peri-implantitis) and demonstrate success and survival rates compared with individuals with a healthy periodontal status (Swierkot et al., 2012). Table 12.2 summarizes the outcome of dental implant therapy in patients with treated GAgP.

Discussion

It has been emphasized that neglected or poorly treated periodontitis increases the risk for peri-implant diseases (Leonhardt et al., 2002). It has also been suggested that patients should not be subjected to dental implant therapy if they present with a poor oral hygiene status and/or oral soft-tissue inflammation (Buser et al., 1990). Therefore, infection control, including extraction of periodontally hopeless teeth, oral hygiene instructions and maintenance, scaling and root planing with or without periodontal surgery should be performed prior to implant placement. The significance of infection control in humans prior to implant therapy has also been supported by results from

Table 12.1 Studies assessing the outcome of dental implant therapy among patients with treated chronic periodontitis.

| Authors et al. (Year) | Study design | Patients with CP / HC | Follow-up | Implant success/survival rate | | Can dental implants osseointegrate and remain functionally stable in patients with treated CP? |
				Implant success/survival rate in patients with treated CP	Implant success/survival rate in HC	
Watson et al. (1999)	Prospective	7CP/19HC	3–4 years	100%	100%	Yes
Karoussis et al. (2003)	Prospective	8CP/45HC	10 years	52.4%	79.1%	No
Evian et al. (2004)	Retrospective	77CP/72HP	~2.5 years	71.2%	91.6%	No
Wennstrom et al. (2004)	Prospective RCT	51CP patients	5 years	NR	NR	Yes
De Boever et al. (2009)	Prospective	68CP/26HC	~4 years	96%	98%	Yes
Roccuzzo et al. (2012)	Prospective	90CP/61HC	10 years	72.8%	93.4%	No
Roccuzzo et al. (2014)	Prospective	45CP/32HC	10 years	100%	97.1%	Yes

CP: Chronic periodontitis
HC: Healthy controls
NR: Not reported

Table 12.2 Studies assessing the outcome of dental implant therapy among patients with treated generalized aggressive periodontitis.

| Authors et al. (Year) | Study design | Patients with GAgP / HC | Follow-up | Implant success/survival rate | | Can dental implants osseointegrate and remain functionally stable in patients with treated GAgP? |
				Implant success/survival rate in patients with treated GAgP	Implant success/survival rate in HC	
Mengel et al. (2001)	Prospective	5GAgP/NR	5 years	88.8%	NR	Yes
Mengel et al. (2005)	Prospective	15GAgP/12HC	3 years	97.8%	100%	Yes
Mengel et al. (2007)	Prospective	5GAgP/5HC	10 years	83.3%	100%	Yes
De Boever et al. (2009)	Prospective	16GAgP/26HC	~4 years	80%	98%	No
Swierkot et al. (2012)	Prospective	35GAgP/18HC	15 years	96%	100%	No

CP: Chronic periodontitis
HC: Healthy controls
NR: Not reported

studies on animal models (Berglundh et al., 1992; Ericsson et al., 1992; Abrahamsson et al., 1998). This suggests that the success and survival of dental implants is not compromised as long as implant therapy is performed after treatment of CP and GAgP. Moreover, routine oral hygiene maintenance and regular follow-up may also play a role in the long-term success and survival of dental implants among patients with a history of CP and GAgP. Implant placement in freshly extraction sockets and immediate loading may be an alternative treatment option.

> **Conclusion**
>
> Dental implants can osseointegrate and remain functionally stable in patients with a history of periodontitis.
>
> GRADE ACCORDING TO LEVEL OF EVIDENCE: **B**

References

Abrahamsson, I., Berglundh, T. and Lindhe, J. 1998. Soft tissue response to plaque formation at different implant systems. A comparative study in the dog. *Clinical Oral Implants Research* 9, pp. 73–79.

Albandar, J. M. and Tinoco, E. M. 2002. Global epidemiology of periodontal diseases in children and young persons. *Periodontology* 2000 29, pp. 153–176.

Berglundh, T., Lindhe, J., Marinello, C., Ericsson, I. and Liljenberg, B. 1992. Soft tissue reaction to de novo plaque formation on implants and teeth. An experimental study in the dog. *Clinical Oral Implants Research* 3, pp. 1–8.

Boutin, S., Hagenfeld, D., Zimmermann, H., El Sayed, N., Hopker, T., Greiser, H. K., Becher, H., Kim, T. S. and Dalpke, A. H. 2017. Clustering of subgingival microbiota reveals microbial disease ecotypes associated with clinical stages of periodontitis in a cross-sectional study. *Frontiers in Microbiology* 8, pp. 340.

Buser, D., Weber, H. P. and Bragger, U. 1990. The treatment of partially edentulous patients with iti hollow-screw implants: Presurgical evaluation and surgical procedures. *The International Journal of Oral & Maxillofacial Implants* 5, pp. 165–175.

De Boever, A. L., Quirynen, M., Coucke, W., Theuniers, G. and De Boever, J. A. 2009. Clinical and radiographic study of implant treatment outcome in periodontally susceptible and non-susceptible patients: A prospective long-term study. *Clinical Oral Implants Research* 20, pp. 1341–1350.

Dingsdag, S., Nelson, S. and Coleman, N. V. 2016. Bacterial communities associated with apical periodontitis and dental implant failure. *Microbial Ecology in Health and Disease* 27, pp. 31307.

Deepti, Tewari, S., Narula, S. C., Singhal, S. R. and Sharma, R. K. 2017. Effect of non-surgical periodontal therapy along with myo-inositol on high-sensitivity c-reactive protein and insulin resistance in women with polycystic ovary syndrome and chronic periodontitis: A randomized controlled trial. *Journal of Periodontology* 88(10): 999–1011. doi: 10.1902/jop.2017.170121.

Ericsson, I., Berglundh, T., Marinello, C., Liljenberg, B. and Lindhe, J. 1992. Long-standing plaque and gingivitis at implants and teeth in the dog. *Clinical Oral Implants Research* 3, pp. 99–103.

Evian, C. I., Emling, R., Rosenberg, E. S., Waasdorp, J. A., Halpern, W., Shah, S. and Garcia, M. 2004. Retrospective analysis of implant survival and the influence of periodontal disease and immediate placement on long-term results. *The International Journal of Oral & Maxillofacial Implants* 19, pp. 393–398.

Greenstein, G., Cavallaro, J., Jr. and Tarnow, D. 2010. Dental implants in the periodontal patient. *Dental Clinics of North America* 54, pp. 113–128.

Heitz-Mayfield, L. J. 2008. Peri-implant diseases: Diagnosis and risk indicators. *Journal of Clinical Periodontology* 35, pp. 292–304.

Karoussis, I. K., Salvi, G. E., Heitz-Mayfield, L. J., Bragger, U., Hammerle, C. H. and Lang, N. P. 2003. Long-term implant prognosis in patients with and without a history of chronic periodontitis: A 10-year prospective cohort study of the iti dental implant system. *Clinical Oral Implants Research* 14, pp. 329–339.

Klinge, B. and Meyle, J. 2012. Peri-implant tissue destruction. The third eao consensus conference 2012. *Clinical Oral Implants Research* 23 Suppl 6, pp. 108–110.

Leonhardt, A., Grondahl, K., Bergstrom, C. and Lekholm, U. 2002. Long-term follow-up of osseointegrated titanium implants using clinical, radiographic and microbiological parameters. *Clinical Oral Implants Research* 13, pp. 127–132.

Lindhe, J., Berglundh, T., Ericsson, I., Liljenberg, B. and Marinello, C. 1992. Experimental breakdown of peri-implant and periodontal tissues. A study in the beagle dog. *Clinical Oral Implants Research* 3, pp. 9–16.

Mengel, R., Schroder, T. and Flores-de-Jacoby, L. 2001. Osseointegrated implants in patients treated for generalized chronic periodontitis and generalized aggressive periodontitis: 3- and 5-year results of a prospective long-term study. *Journal of Periodontology* 72, pp. 977–989.

Mengel, R. and Flores-de-Jacoby, L. 2005. Implants in patients treated for generalized aggressive and chronic periodontitis: A 3-year prospective longitudinal study. *Journal of Periodontology* 76, pp. 534–543.

Mengel, R., Behle, M. and Flores-de-Jacoby, L. 2007. Osseointegrated implants in subjects treated for generalized aggressive periodontitis: 10-year results of a prospective, long-term cohort study. *Journal of Periodontology* 78, pp. 2229–2237.

Mombelli, A., van Oosten, M. A., Schurch, E., Jr. and Land, N. P. 1987. The microbiota associated with successful or failing osseointegrated titanium implants. *Oral Microbiology and Immunology* 2, pp. 145–151.

Monje, A., Alcoforado, G., Padial-Molina, M., Suarez, F., Lin, G. H. and Wang, H. L. 2014. Generalized aggressive periodontitis as a risk factor for dental implant failure: A systematic review and meta-analysis. *Journal of Periodontology* 85, pp. 1398–1407.

Ong, C. T., Ivanovski, S., Needleman, I. G., Retzepi, M., Moles, D. R., Tonetti, M. S. and Donos, N. 2008. Systematic review of implant outcomes in treated periodontitis subjects. *Journal of Clinical Periodontology* 35, pp. 438–462.

Paster, B. J., Boches, S. K., Galvin, J. L., Ericson, R. E., Lau, C. N., Levanos, V. A., Sahasrabudhe, A. and Dewhirst, F. E. 2001. Bacterial diversity in human subgingival plaque. *Journal of Bacteriology* 183, pp. 3770–3783.

Roccuzzo, M., Bonino, L., Dalmasso, P. and Aglietta, M. 2014. Long-term results of a three arms prospective cohort study on implants in periodontally compromised patients: 10-year data around sandblasted and acid-etched (sla) surface. *Clinical Oral Implants Research* 25, pp. 1105–1112.

Romanos, G. E., Javed, F., Delgado-Ruiz, R. A. and Calvo-Guirado, J. L. 2015. Peri-implant diseases: A review of treatment interventions. *Dental Clinics of North America* 59, pp. 157–178.

Roos-Jansaker, A. M., Lindahl, C., Renvert, H. and Renvert, S. 2006a. Nine- to fourteen-year follow-up of implant treatment. Part i: Implant loss and associations to various factors. *Journal of Clinical Periodontology* 33, pp. 283–289.

Roos-Jansaker, A. M., Renvert, H., Lindahl, C. and Renvert, S. 2006b. Nine- to fourteen-year follow-up of implant treatment. Part iii: Factors associated with peri-implant lesions. *Journal of Clinical Periodontology* 33, pp. 296–301.

Safii, S. H., Palmer, R. M. and Wilson, R. F. 2010. Risk of implant failure and marginal bone loss in subjects with a history of periodontitis: A systematic review and meta-analysis. *Clinical Implant Dentistry and Related Research* 12, pp. 165–174.

Swierkot, K., Lottholz, P., Flores-de-Jacoby, L. and Mengel, R. 2012. Mucositis, peri-implantitis, implant success, and survival of implants in patients with treated generalized aggressive periodontitis: 3- to 16-year results of a prospective long-term cohort study. *Journal of Periodontology* 83, pp. 1213–1225.

Watson, C. J., Tinsley, D., Ogden, A. R., Russell, J. L., Mulay, S. and Davison, E. M. 1999. A 3- to 4-year study of single tooth hydroxylapatite coated endosseous dental implants. *British Dental Journal* 187, pp. 90–94.

13

Success and Survival of Dental Implants during Pregnancy

Introduction

During pregnancy, imbalances in sex hormones affect various organs and produce alterations in the immune system (Brabin, 1985; Gursoy et al., 2010; Kovats, 2012). Moreover, there is a reduction in the chemotactic and phagocytic function of neutrophils, inhibition of T-cell activity, and decrease in antibody production (Zachariasen, 1993; Priddy, 1997). Evidence has shown that gingival inflammation is often manifested during the second and third trimester of gestation (Suresh and Radfar, 2004; Gonzalez-Jaranay et al., 2017). One explanation for this is that gingival tissues are influenced by physiological changes in serum concentrations of female sex hormones during gestation, which produces some degree of gingival edema and gingivitis (Figuero et al., 2013). The prevalence of periodontopathogenic microorganisms, such as *Porphyromonas gingivalis*, are frequently present in the oral cavity of pregnant versus nonpregnant females (Kornman and Loesche, 1980). Furthermore, gestational diabetes is also a risk factor for periodontal disease during pregnancy (Abariga and Whitcomb, 2016).

Results

Results from a clinical study showed that the percentage of sites with probing depth >3 mm were higher in pregnant females throughout the pregnancy phase compared with postpartum (Gonzalez-Jaranay et al., 2017). In this context, attention of oral health care providers may be warranted as a result of the multiple physiologic/hormonal changes associated with pregnancy. This suggests that the prevalence of peri-implant diseases, such as peri-implant mucositis and peri-implantitis, are significantly higher among pregnant versus nonpregnant women. However, upon a vigilant review of indexed literature, no studies assessing the success and/or survival rate of dental implants in pregnant females were identified (Table 13.1). Hence, further research is needed in this area.

Table 13.1 Peri-implant status in pregnant females.

Authors et al.	Mean age	Trimester	Implant dimensions	Jaw location	Peri-implant plaque index	Peri-implant bleeding on probing	Peri-implant probing depth	Peri-implant marginal bone loss

There are no studies in indexed literature.

Evidence-based Implant Dentistry and Systemic Conditions, First Edition.
Fawad Javed and Georgios E. Romanos.
© 2018 John Wiley & Sons, Inc. Published 2018 by John Wiley & Sons, Inc.

> **Conclusion**
>
> There is no evidence regarding the success and survival of dental implants in pregnant females. Hence, further studies are warranted in this regard.
>
> GRADE ACCORDING TO LEVEL OF EVIDENCE: **E**

References

Abariga, S. A., & Whitcomb, B. W. 2016. Periodontitis and gestational diabetes mellitus: a systematic review and meta-analysis of observational studies. *BMC Pregnancy Childbirth* 16, p. 344. doi:10.1186/s12884-016-1145-z.

Brabin, B. J. 1985. Epidemiology of infection in pregnancy. *Rev Infect Dis* 7, pp. 579–603.

Figuero, E., Carrillo-de-Albornoz, A., Martin, C., Tobias, A., & Herrera, D. 2013. Effect of pregnancy on gingival inflammation in systemically healthy women: a systematic review. *Journal of Clinical Periodontology* 40, pp. 457–473. doi:10.1111/jcpe.12053.

Gonzalez-Jaranay, M., Tellez, L., Roa-Lopez, A., Gomez-Moreno, G., & Moreu, G. 2017. Periodontal status during pregnancy and postpartum. *PLoS One* 12, pp. e0178234. doi:10.1371/journal.pone.0178234.

Gursoy, M., Kononen, E., Tervahartiala, T., Gursoy, U. K., Pajukanta, R., & Sorsa, T. 2010. Longitudinal study of salivary proteinases during pregnancy and postpartum. *Journal of Periodontal Research* 45, pp. 496–503. doi:10.1111/j.1600-0765.2009.01264.x.

Kornman, K. S., & Loesche, W. J. 1980. The subgingival microbial flora during pregnancy. *Journal of Periodontal Research* 15, pp. 111–122.

Kovats, S. 2012. Estrogen receptors regulate an inflammatory pathway of dendritic cell differentiation: mechanisms and implications for immunity. *Hormones and Behavior* 62, pp. 254–262. doi:10.1016/j.yhbeh.2012.04.011.

Priddy, K. D. 1997. Immunologic adaptations during pregnancy. *Journal of Obstetric, Gynecologic, and Neonatal Nursing* 26, pp. 388–394.

Suresh, L., & Radfar, L. 2004. Pregnancy and lactation. *Oral Surgery, Oral Medicine, Oral Pathology, Oral Radiology, and Endodontology* 97, pp. 672–682. doi:10.1016/s1079210404000861.

Zachariasen, R. D. 1993. The effect of elevated ovarian hormones on periodontal health: oral contraceptives and pregnancy. *Women Health* 20, pp. 21–30. doi:10.1300/J013v20n02_02.

14

Dental Implants in Patients with Psychological/Psychiatric Disorders

Introduction: Periodontal Health Status among Patients with Psychological/Psychiatric Disorders

It has been reported that scores of periodontal inflammatory parameters (including bleeding on probing, probing depth, and dental calculus index) are poorer among patients with psychiatric disorders, such as schizophrenia and mood disorders (Nayak et al., 2016). *Porphyromonas gingivalis* (*P. gingivalis*) (a classical microbe associated with the etiology of periodontal disease) can transmigrate to the brain and modulate an innate inflammatory response (Harding et al., 2017). In patients with Alzheimer's disease, *P. gingivalis* inhibits the local interferon-gamma response by preventing entry of immune cells into the brain (Ide et al., 2016). Moreover, an increased number of missing teeth has also been associated with an increased incidence and prevalence of dementia (Stein et al., 2007).

Hypothesis

Since patients with psychological/psychiatric disorders are more susceptible to periodontal disease (Stein et al., 2007; Nayak et al., 2016); it is hypothesized that the outcome of dental implant therapy is compromised in patients with psychological/psychiatric disorders as compared to healthy individuals.

Objective

The aim of this chapter to review indexed literature to determine whether dental implants can remain functionally stable in patients with psychological/psychiatric disorders.

Materials and Methods

Eligibility Criteria

The following eligibility criteria were entailed: (a) clinical studies and (b) placement and survival of dental implants in animals or human patients with psychological/psychiatric disorders. Literature reviews, letters to the editor, and commentaries were excluded.

Evidence-based Implant Dentistry and Systemic Conditions, First Edition.
Fawad Javed and Georgios E. Romanos.
© 2018 John Wiley & Sons, Inc. Published 2018 by John Wiley & Sons, Inc.

Literature Search

PubMed/Medline (National Library of Medicine, Bethesda, Maryland), EMBASE, ISI-Web of Knowledge, SCOPUS, and Google-Scholar databases were searched up to March 2017 using the following key words in different combinations: "dementia," "dental implant," "failure," "Alzheimer's disease," "psychological," "psychiatric," "survival," and "success." Titles and abstracts of studies that fulfilled the eligibility criteria were screened and checked for agreement. Full texts of studies judged by title and abstract to be relevant were read and assessed in accordance with the eligibility criteria (as previously stated). In addition, hand searching of the reference lists of potentially relevant original and review studies was also performed and checked for agreement via discussion.

Results

A limited number of studies have assessed the success and survival of dental implants in patients with psychological/psychiatric disorders (Kromminga et al., 1991; Griess et al., 1998; Ekfeldt et al., 2001; Tinner and Marinello, 2002; Kubo and Kimura, 2004; Addy et al., 2006). In the retrospective study, personal grief and depression were nominated as significant risk factors associated with dental implant failure (Ekfeldt et al., 2001). In the study by Addy, Korszun, and Jagger (2006), dental implant-retained prostheses were provided to three patients with psychiatric disorders. The study concluded that psychiatric disorders are not a contraindication to dental implant therapy (Addy et al., 2006). Results from a five-year follow-up study showed that a dental implant-retained prosthesis can remain functionally stable in patients with schizophrenia (Griess et al., 1998). Similarly, results from another case-report showed successful implant surgery in the maxilla in a 72-year-old patient with Parkinson's disease; however, follow-up results were not reported in this study (Kubo and Kimura, 2004). On the contrary, another case-report, Kromminga et al. (1991) concluded that outcomes of dental implant therapy are compromised among patients with psychological disorders.

Discussion

The literature with respect to the success and survival of dental implants in patients with psychiatric/psychological diseases is sparse and inconsistent. However, poor oral hygiene status, oral para-functional habits such as bruxism, habits such as repeated insertion of fingers in the mouth, and behavioral issues are common in patients with psychiatric/psychological diseases. Such factors may complicate dental implant therapy in these patients and jeopardize the long-term success and survival of dental implants.

Conclusion
There is insufficient evidence to determine whether, in the long-term, dental implants can remain functionally stable in patients with psychological/psychiatric disorders. Hence, further studies are warranted in this regard.
GRADE ACCORDING TO LEVEL OF EVIDENCE: **D**

References

Addy, L., Korszun, A. and Jagger, R. G. 2006. Dental implant treatment for patients with psychiatric disorders. *European Journal of Prosthodontics and Restorative Dentistry* 14, pp. 90–92.

Ekfeldt, A., Christiansson, U., Eriksson, T., Linden, U., Lundqvist, S., Rundcrantz, T., Johansson, L. A., Nilner, K. and Billstrom, C. 2001. A retrospective analysis of factors associated with multiple implant failures in maxillae. *Clinical Oral Implants Research* 12, pp. 462–467.

Griess, M., Reilmann, B. and Chanavaz, M. 1998. The multi-modal prosthetic treatment of mentally handicapped patients – necessity and challenge. *European Journal of Prosthodontics and Restorative Dentistry* 6, pp. 115–120.

Harding, A., Robinson, S., Crean, S. and Singhrao, S. K. 2017. Can better management of periodontal disease delay the onset and progression of Alzheimer's disease? *Journal of Alzheimers Disease*. doi:10.3233/jad-170046.

Ide, M., Harris, M., Stevens, A., Sussams, R., Hopkins, V., Culliford, D., Fuller, J., Ibbett, P., Raybould, R., Thomas, R., Puenter, U., Teeling, J., Perry, V. H. and Holmes, C. 2016. Periodontitis and cognitive decline in Alzheimer's disease. *PLoS One* 11, pp. e0151081. doi:10.1371/journal.pone.0151081.

Kromminga, R., Habel, G. and Muller-Fahlbusch, H. 1991. [Failure of dental implants following psychosomatic disturbances in the stomatognathic system – a clinical-catamnestic study]. *Dtsch Stomatol* 41, pp. 233–236.

Kubo, K. and Kimura, K. 2004. Implant surgery for a patient with Parkinson's disease controlled by intravenous midazolam: a case report. *The International Journal of Oral & Maxillofacial Implants* 19, pp. 288–290.

Nayak, S. U., Singh, R. and Kota, K. P. 2016. Periodontal Health among Non-Hospitalized Chronic Psychiatric Patients in Mangaluru City-India. *Journal of Clinical Diagnostic Research* 10, pp. Zc40–43. doi:10.7860/jcdr/2016/19501.8248.

Stein, P. S., Desrosiers, M., Donegan, S. J., Yepes, J. F. and Kryscio, R. J. 2007. Tooth loss, dementia and neuropathology in the Nun study. *Journal of the American Dental Association* 138, pp. 1314–1322; quiz 1381–1312.

Tinner, D. and Marinello, C. P. 2002. [Implant-supported dental prostheses in a depressed patient-a case report]. *Schweiz Monatsschr Zahnmed* 112, pp. 495–507.

15

Dental Implants in Patients Using Recreational Drugs

Introduction

Recreational drugs are psychoactive drugs that alter a person' mental state in a way that modifies emotions, perceptions, and feelings for recreational purposes. Recreational drugs that have been classified as controlled and illegal vary by country, but they usually include cannabis, methamphetamines, heroin, cocaine, marijuana, and hashish. Habitual use of recreational drugs has been associated with complications including myocardial infarction and necrosis, renal amyloidosis, preterm delivery, and sudden death (Fineschi et al., 1997; Manner et al., 2009; Fischbach, 2017; Maghsoudlou et al., 2017).

Results

A recent study investigated the association between cocaine addiction and dental health (Cury et al., 2017). In this study, 40 cocaine-addicted men and 120 controls (nonaddicted men) aged at least 18 years underwent a full-mouth decayed, missing, and filled teeth (DMFT) examination. The results showed a positive association between decayed teeth and cocaine addiction; whereas, filled and missing teeth showed a negative association (Cury et al., 2017). Another study showed that probing depth is significantly higher in cocaine-addicted individuals compared to nonaddicted controls (Cury et al., 2017). Moreover, habitual use of recreational drugs has been associated with an increased prevalence of residual roots, gingivitis, and gingival necrosis (Gariulo et al., 1985; Ma et al., 2012). It is therefore likely that the prevalence of peri-implant diseases (peri-implant mucositis and peri-implantitis) are also significantly higher among recreational drug users compared with nonaddicted controls. However, upon an exhaustive search of indexed literature, no studies assessing the impact of habitual recreational drug use on peri-implant inflammatory parameters such as plaque index, gingival index, probing depth, and crestal bone loss were identified (Table 15.1).

Evidence-based Implant Dentistry and Systemic Conditions, First Edition.
Fawad Javed and Georgios E. Romanos.
© 2018 John Wiley & Sons, Inc. Published 2018 by John Wiley & Sons, Inc.

Table 15.1 Studies assessing the clinical and radiographic peri-implant inflammatory parameters among habitual recreational drug users.

Authors et al. (Year)	Study design	Participants	Type of recreational drug used	Duration of habit	Daily frequency of recreational drug use	Peri-implant plaque index	Peri-implant bleeding on probing	Peri-implant probing depth	Peri-implant crestal bone loss

There are no studies in indexed literature.

> **Conclusion**
>
> The impact of habitual use of recreational drugs on the success and survival of dental implants remains unknown. Further long-term follow-up studies are needed in this regard.
>
> GRADE ACCORDING TO LEVEL OF EVIDENCE: **E**

References

Cury, P. R., Oliveira, M. G., de Andrade, K. M., de Freitas, M. D. and Dos Santos, J. N. 2017. Dental health status in crack/cocaine-addicted men: A cross-sectional study. *Environmental science and pollution research international* 24, pp. 7585–7590.

Cury, P. R., Oliveira, M. G. and Dos Santos, J. N. 2017. Periodontal status in crack and cocaine addicted men: A cross-sectional study. *Environmental Science and Pollution Research International* 24, pp. 3423–3429.

Fineschi, V., Wetli, C. V., Di Paolo, M. and Baroldi, G. 1997. Myocardial necrosis and cocaine. A quantitative morphologic study in 26 cocaine-associated deaths. *International Journal of Legal Medicine* 110, pp. 193–198.

Fischbach, P. 2017. The role of illicit drug use in sudden death in the young. *Cardiology in the Young* 27, pp. S75–s79.

Gariulo, A. V., Jr., Toto, P. D. and Gargiulo, A. W. 1985. Cocaine induced-gingival necrosis. *Periodontal Case Reports : A Publication of the Northeastern Society of Periodontists* 7, pp. 44–45.

Ma, H., Shi, X. C., Hu, D. Y. and Li, X. 2012. The poor oral health status of former heroin users treated with methadone in a chinese city. *Medical Science Monitor: International Medical Journal of Experimental and Clinical Research* 18, pp. Ph51–55.

Maghsoudlou, S., Cnattingius, S., Montgomery, S., Aarabi, M., Semnani, S., Wikstrom, A. K. and Bahmanyar, S. 2017. Opium use during pregnancy and risk of preterm delivery: A population-based cohort study. *PloS One* 12, pp. e0176588.

Manner, I., Sagedal, S., Roger, M. and Os, I. 2009. Renal amyloidosis in intravenous heroin addicts with nephrotic syndrome and renal failure. *Clinical Nephrology* 72, pp. 224–228.

16

Dental Implants in Patients with Renal Disorders

Introduction

Periodontal Health Status among Patients with Renal Disorders

The association between periodontal disease (PD) and renal disorders remains debatable. Studies have shown that there is a higher prevalence of renal disorders (such as chronic kidney disease [CKD] and end-stage renal disease [ESRD]) among patients with periodontal disease (PD) compared with individuals without PD (Ismail et al., 2013; Limeres et al., 2016). Similarly, Yoshihara et al. (2017) suggested that periodontal inflammation is associated with poor renal function. However, controversial results have also been reported. In the study by Castillo et al. (2007), there was no statistically significant association between PD and ESRD.

Impact of Renal Diseases on Osseointegration

The effect on osseointegration remain poorly investigated among patients with chronic kidney disease (CKD) remain poorly understood. Histomorphometric results from an experimental study on mice showed significantly lower bone-to-implant contact ratio at two weeks of healing in mice with CKD compared with mice in the control-groups (mice without CKD) (Zou et al., 2013). In another experimental study, titanium implants were inserted in the distal end of the femurs in mice with and without induced CKD (Sun et al., 2015). The mouse model was treated with fibroblast growth factor (FGF)-23 neutralizing antibody to assess its effect bone structure and implant fixation. The results showed that FGF-23 neutralization significantly improved the strength of osseointegration, as evidenced by a biomechanical push-in test (Sun et al., 2015). Similar results were reported in another experimental study (Liu et al., 2014).

Hypothesis

Since results from experimental studies have shown that it is possible to achieve osseointegration in animals with induced CKD (Zou et al., 2013; Liu et al., 2014; Sun et al., 2015), it is hypothesized that dental implants can osseointegrate and remain functionally stable in patients with renal disorders.

Evidence-based Implant Dentistry and Systemic Conditions, First Edition.
Fawad Javed and Georgios E. Romanos.
© 2018 John Wiley & Sons, Inc. Published 2018 by John Wiley & Sons, Inc.

Objective

The aim of this chapter is to review indexed literature to determine whether dental implants can remain functionally stable in patients with renal disorders.

Materials and Methods

Eligibility Criteria

The following eligibility criteria were entailed: (a) clinical and experimental studies and (b) placement and survival of dental implants in animals or human patients with renal disorders. Literature reviews, letters to the editor, commentaries, and articles published in languages other than English were excluded.

Literature Search

PubMed/Medline (National Library of Medicine, Bethesda, Maryland), EMBASE, ISI-Web of Knowledge, SCOPUS, and Google-Scholar databases were searched up to February 2018 using the following key words in different combinations: "chronic kidney disease," "dental implant," "hemodialysis," "end-stage renal disease," "survival," and "success." Titles and abstracts of studies that fulfilled the eligibility criteria were screened and checked for agreement. Full texts of studies judged by title and abstract to be relevant were read and assessed in accordance with the eligibility criteria (as stated above). In addition, hand searching of the reference lists of potentially relevant original and review studies was also performed and checked for agreement via discussion.

Results

Five studies were included and processed for data extraction (Zou et al., 2013; Liu et al., 2014; Flanagan and Mancini, 2015; Sun et al., 2015; Zhang et al., 2015). Four studies (Zou et al., 2013; Liu et al., 2014; Sun et al., 2015; Zhang et al., 2015) were performed in mice with CKD and one study was a case-report based on a 32-year-old male patient with renal failure (RF) (Flanagan and Mancini, 2015). Histomorphometric results by Zhang et al. (2015) showed that estrogen deficiency has a synergistic effect with CKD and impaired BIC ratio and implant push-in resistance in mice with CKD. Other experimental studies showed that adjunct therapies such as vitamin D supplementation and fibroblast growth factor-23 neutralizing antibody injections enhanced the strength of osseointegration, as evidenced by a biomechanical push-in test in CKD mice (Liu et al., 2014; Sun et al., 2015). Two-year follow-up results from the only case-report included in this chapter showed that dental implants can remain functionally stable in patients with renal RF (Flanagan and Mancini, 2015). These results are summarized in Table 16.1.

Discussion

It is tempting to speculate that dental implants can osseointegrate and remain functionally stable in patients with renal disorders; however, the outcomes of implant therapy as reported in this chapter should be interpreted with caution. This is primarily due to the

Table 16.1 Outcomes of studies assessing the success and survival of dental implants in patients with renal disorders.

Authors et al. (year)	Study design	Study subjects	Location of implant	Study groups	Duration of study	Outcome
Zou et al. (2013)	Experimental	Mice	Femur	Test-group: mice with CKD Control-group: mice without CKD	12 weeks	BIC ratio was similar in both groups. Strength of osseointegration, as evidenced by a biomechanical push-in test was significantly higher in the control group.
Liu et al. (2014)	Experimental	Mice	Femur	Test-group: CKD mice with vitamin D supplementation Control-group: CKD mice with vehicle supplementation	12 weeks	BIC ratio and bone volume around the implant were significantly higher in the test-group. Strength of osseointegration, as evidenced by a biomechanical push-in test, was significantly higher in the test group.
Flanagan and Mancini (2015)	Case-report	Long-term dialysis patient with CKD	Maxilla	NA	2 years	Dental implants can osseointegrate and remain functionally stable in patients with CKD.
Sun et al. (2015)	Experimental	Mice with CKD	Tibia	Test-group: FGF-23 neutralizing antibody injection Control-group: sham injection	12 weeks	BIC ratio was similar in both groups. Strength of osseointegration, as evidenced by a biomechanical push-in test, was significantly higher in the test-group.
Zhang et al. (2015)	Experimental	Mice	Femur	Test-group: mice with CKD and OVX Control-group: mice without CKD and OVX	12 weeks	Estrogen deficiency has a synergistic effect with CKD, impaired BIC ratio and implant push-in resistance in mice with CKD.

BIC: Bone-to-implant
CKD: Chronic kidney disease
FGF: Fibroblast growth factor
NA: Not applicable
OVX: Ovariectomy

fact that 80% of the studies included were performed on animal-models with induced CKD (Zou et al., 2013; Liu et al., 2014; Sun et al., 2015; Zhang et al., 2015). However, it is proposed that a timely diagnosis and management of renal diseases (with treatments such as vitamin D supplementation) may contribute toward the success and survival of dental implants in these patients.

It is also pertinent to mention that patient compliance (toward dietary control as well as regular oral hygiene maintenance) is an essential parameter that plays an essential role in the success and survival of dental implants in medically compromised individuals (Al Amri et al., 2016). In the case-report by Flanagan and Mancini (2015), the patient has a history of noncompliance. The patient was counseled on this issue as this factor may affect the durability and long-term outcome of the implant therapy. The patient agreed to comply with the instructions (dietary restrictions) provided by the operators. This could be an explanation for the two-year follow-up outcome of this case-report according to which dental implants remained functionally stable in this patient. This reflects that besides other factors such as systemic health and bone quality, patient education and compliance also play a role in the long-term success and survival of dental implants.

Conclusion

There is insufficient evidence to determine whether dental implants can remain functionally stable in the long-term among patients with renal disorders. Hence, further studies are warranted in this regard.

GRADE ACCORDING TO LEVEL OF EVIDENCE: **D**

References

Al Amri, M. D., Kellesarian, S. V., Al-Kheraif, A. A., Malmstrom, H., Javed, F., & Romanos, G. E. 2016. Effect of oral hygiene maintenance on HbA1c levels and peri-implant parameters around immediately-loaded dental implants placed in type-2 diabetic patients: 2 years follow-up. *Clinical Oral Implants Research* 27, pp. 1439–1443. doi:10.1111/clr.12758.

Castillo, A., Mesa, F., Liebana, J., Garcia-Martinez, O., Ruiz, S., Garcia-Valdecasas, J., & O'Valle, F. 2007. Periodontal and oral microbiological status of an adult population undergoing haemodialysis: a cross-sectional study. *Oral Diseases* 13, pp. 198–205. doi:10.1111/j.1601-0825.2006.01267.x.

Flanagan, D. & Mancini, M. 2015. Bimaxillary full arch fixed dental implant supported treatment for a patient with renal failure and secondary hyperparathyroidism and osteodystrophy. *Journal of Oral Implantology* 41, pp. e36–43. doi:10.1563/aaid-joi-d-13-00188.

Ismail, G., Dumitriu, H. T., Dumitriu, A. S., & Ismail, F. B. 2013. Periodontal disease: a covert source of inflammation in chronic kidney disease patients. *International Journal of Nephrology* 2013, pp. 515796. doi:10.1155/2013/515796.

Limeres, J., Garcez, J. F., Marinho, J. S., Loureiro, A., Diniz, M., & Diz, P. 2016. Early tooth loss in end-stage renal disease patients on haemodialysis. *Oral Diseases* 22, pp. 530–535. doi:10.1111/odi.12486.

Liu, W., Zhang, S., Zhao, D., Zou, H., Sun, N., Liang, X., Dard, M., Lanske, B. & Yuan, Q. 2014. Vitamin D supplementation enhances the fixation of titanium implants in chronic kidney disease in mice. *PLoS One* 9, pp. e95689. doi:10.1371/journal.pone.0095689.

Sun, N., Guo, Y., Liu, W., Densmore, M., Shalhoub, V., Erben, R. G., Ye, L., Lanske, B., & Yuan, Q. 2015. FGF23 neutralization improves bone quality and osseointegration of titanium implants in chronic kidney disease mice. *Scientific Reports* 5, pp. 8304. fdoi:10.1038/srep08304.

Yoshihara, A., Sugita, N., Iwasaki, M., Wang, Y., Miyazaki, H., Yoshie, H., & Nakamura, K. 2017. Relationship between renal function and periodontal disease in community-dwelling elderly women with different genotypes. *Journal of Clinical Periodontology* doi:10.1111/jcpe.12708.

Zhang, S., Guo, Y., Zou, H., Sun, N., Zhao, D., Liu, W., Dong, Y., Cheng, G., & Yuan, Q. 2015. Effect of estrogen deficiency on the fixation of titanium implants in chronic kidney disease mice. *Osteoporos International* 26, pp. 1073–1080. doi:10.1007/s00198-014-2952-6.

Zou, H., Zhao, X., Sun, N., Zhang, S., Sato, T., Yu, H., Chen, Q., Weber, H. P., Dard, M., Yuan, Q., & Lanske, B. 2013. Effect of chronic kidney disease on the healing of titanium implants. *Bone* 56, pp. 410–415. doi:10.1016/j.bone.2013.07.014.

17

Dental Implants in Patients with Rheumatic Diseases

Introduction

Rheumatic diseases (RD) (synonym: musculoskeletal diseases) are characterized by pain and reduction in the range of function and motion in one or more areas of the musculo-skeletal system. RD include over 200 different diseases, which span from various types of arthritis to osteoporosis and on to systemic connective tissue diseases. In some forms of rheumatic diseases, there are signs of inflammation such as swelling, redness, and warmth in the affected areas. RD affect individuals in all age groups and both genders; however, females are more frequently affected than males. Some common risk factors of RD include advancing age, overweight and obesity, tobacco smoking, and genetic factors (Choi, 2005; Clarke and Vyse, 2009; Kallberg et al., 2011; Gremese et al., 2014).

Hypothesis

It is hypothesized that dental implants can osseointegrate and remain functionally stable in patients with RD.

Objective

The aim of this chapter is to review indexed literature to determine whether or not dental implants can remain functionally stable in patients with RD.

Materials and Methods

Eligibility Criteria

The following eligibility criteria were entailed: (a) clinical studies and (b) placement and survival of dental implants in animals or human patients with rheumatological disorders. Literature reviews, experimental studies, letters to the editor, commentaries and articles published in languages other than English were excluded.

Evidence-based Implant Dentistry and Systemic Conditions, First Edition.
Fawad Javed and Georgios E. Romanos.
© 2018 John Wiley & Sons, Inc. Published 2018 by John Wiley & Sons, Inc.

Literature Search

PubMed/Medline (National Library of Medicine, Bethesda, Maryland), EMBASE, ISI-Web of Knowledge, SCOPUS, and Google-Scholar databases were searched up to February 2018 using the following key words in different combinations: "arthritis," "rheumatological disorders," "dental implant," "osteoarthritis," "rheumatoid arthritis," "survival," and "success." Titles and abstracts of studies that fulfilled the eligibility criteria were screened and checked for agreement. Full texts of studies judged by title and abstract to be relevant were read and assessed in accordance with the eligibility criteria (as previously stated). In addition, hand searching of the reference lists of potentially relevant original and review studies was also performed and checked for agreement via discussion.

Results

Osteoporosis

Osteoporosis is a catabolic bone disease that affects the remodeling of bone and increases their susceptibility to fracture. There is a limited number of clinical studies assessing the success and survival of dental implant placed in patients with osteoporosis. In a recent study (Wagner et al., 2017), the effect of osteoporosis of peri-implant marginal bone remodeling was investigated in post-menopausal osteoporotic females and their respective controls (females without osteoporosis). The implants in both groups had been functional for approximately seven years. The results showed minimal crestal bone loss around implants placed among females with and without osteoporosis with no statistically significant difference between the groups. The authors concluded that osteoporosis is not a contraindication to dental implant therapy (Wagner et al., 2017). Similarly, results from another recent longitudinal study showed that dental implants can remain functionally stable in patients with controlled osteoporosis (Pedro et al., 2017). One-year follow-up results by Temmerman and associates and Siebert and colleagues also showed that dental implant therapy is a suitable therapeutic strategy in patients with osteoporosis (Siebert et al., 2015; Temmerman et al., 2017). A survey study from Toronto assessed whether age and gender (which are known risk-factors of osteoporosis) are also risk factors for patients with dental implants (Dao et al., 1993). In this study (Dao et al., 1993), 36 males and 93 females aged 20–76 years at the time of implant placement, having dental implants in function for 2–11 years were included. The results showed that the highest implant failure rate was seen in individuals below 50 years of age compared with patients over 50 years old. Dao et al. (1993) concluded that patients at risk for osteoporosis are not at risk for implant failure.

It has also been reported that bone regeneration around implants is possible in patients with osteoporosis in a manner similar to systemically healthy individuals (Tadinada et al., 2015). A three-year follow-up study based on a retrospective chart review of patients with and without osteoporosis indicates that a diagnosis of osteoporosis does not contribute to an increased risk of implant failure (Holahan et al., 2008). However, controversial results have also been reported. Results from a clinical study from Germany on 380 patients (including those with osteoporosis) showed that osteoporosis is a statistically significant risk factor for dental implant failure (Niedermaier et al., 2017). Conclusions based on results from a systematic review also showed that rates of implant loss are higher in patients with osteoporosis compared with systemically healthy controls (Giro et al., 2015) (Table 17.1).

Dependent on the treatment of osteoporosis, additional risk factors can be associated with implant failure, especially if patients have a long-term oral or intravenous administration of bisphosphonate therapy (Figures 17.1 to 17.7).

Table 17.1 Outcomes of dental implant therapy in patients with osteoporosis.

Authors et al. (Year)	Study design	Subjects	Follow-up	Outcome	Conclusion
Holahan et al. (2008)	Retrospective	Patients with and without osteoporosis	3 years	There was no statistically significant influence of osteoporosis in peri-implant CBL	Patients with controlled osteoporosis are suitable candidates for dental implant therapy.
Siebert et al. (2105)	Retrospective	Patients with and without osteoporosis	1 year	Implant success rate in patients with osteoporosis was 100%	Patients with controlled osteoporosis are suitable candidates for dental implant therapy.
Tadinada et al. (2015)	Longitudinal	Patients with and without osteoporosis	9 months	CBCT showed evidence of new bone formation in both groups with no statistically significant difference.	Dental implant therapy is a suitable therapeutic strategy in patients with osteoporosis.
Niedermaier et al. (2017)	Retrospective	Study cohort including patients with osteoporosis	7 years	Implant failure was higher in patients with osteoporosis	Osteoporosis is a risk factor for dental implant failure.
Pedro et al. (2017)	Longitudinal	Patients with systemic diseases including osteoporosis	Up to 4 years	There was no statistically significant influence of osteoporosis in peri-implant CBL	Patients with controlled osteoporosis are suitable candidates for dental implant therapy.
Temmerman et al. (2017)	Retrospective	Patients with and without osteoporosis	1 year	There was no statistically significant influence of osteoporosis in peri-implant CBL	Patients with controlled osteoporosis are suitable candidates for dental implant therapy.
Wagner et al. (2017)	Retrospective	Patients with and without osteoporosis	Approximately 7 years in both groups	Minimal CBL around implants in both groups	Patients with controlled osteoporosis are suitable candidates for dental implant therapy.

CBCT: Cone beam computed tomography
CBL: Crestal bone loss

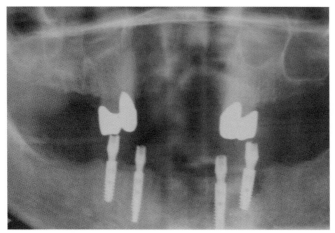

(Surgical Treatment: Dr. D. May, Luenen, Germany)

Figure 17.1 Radiographic evaluation of implants placed in a patient with oral bisphosphonates showing extensive radiolucency at the left side of the mandible.

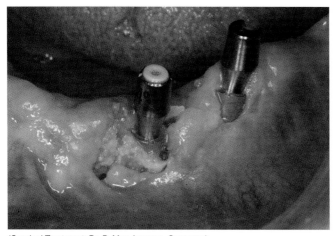

(Surgical Treatment: Dr. D. May, Luenen, Germany)

Figure 17.2 Clinical situation showing the oral bone necrosis around a mandibular implant.

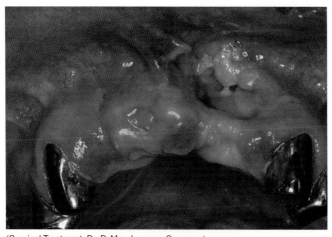

(Surgical Treatment: Dr. D. May, Luenen, Germany)

Figure 17.3 Clinical situation showing the oral bone necrosis in the maxilla of the same patient of the Figure 17.2.

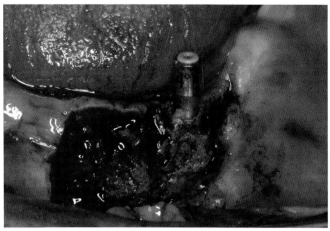

(Surgical Treatment: Dr. D. May, Luenen, Germany)

Figure 17.4 Clinical condition of the necrotic bone at the mandible of a patient with oral bisphosphonates.

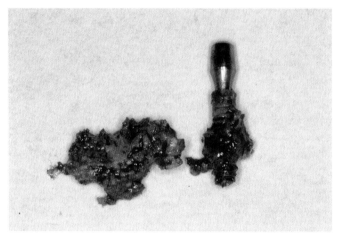

(Surgical Treatment: Dr. D. May, Luenen, Germany)

Figure 17.5 Specimen with the necrotic bone in contact with the implant.

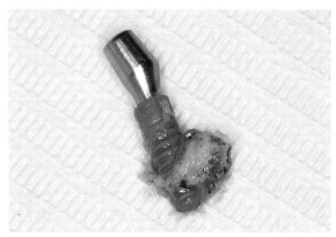

(Surgical Treatment: Dr. D. May, Luenen, Germany)

Figure 17.6 Necrotic bone in contact with the implant, well known as bisphosphonate-associated osteonecrosis of the jaw (BONJ).

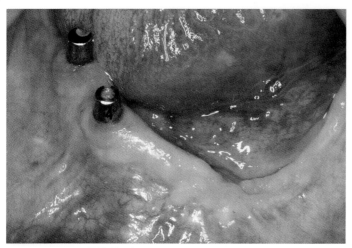

(Surgical Treatment: Dr. D. May, Luenen, Germany)

Figure 17.7 Clinical condition of the mandible after removal of the implants and necrotic bone 2 years after surgery.

Rheumatoid Arthritis

RA is a systemic autoimmune disease characterized by bone damage and chronic synovitis leading to functional disability and morbidity. In a four-year follow-up case-report, Ella and associates placed dental implants in the edentulous maxilla of a 56-year-old female with osteoporosis (Ella et al., 2011). At follow-up, the dental implants remained functionally stable (Ella et al., 2011). Results from the clinical retrospective study showed that dental implants placed in patients with rheumatoid arthritis (RA) can have survival rates of up to 100% (Krennmair et al., 2010). Similar results were reported in a case-series study (Weinlander et al., 2010) (Figures 17.8 to 17.15).

Discussion

From the literature reviewed, it is tempting to conclude that RD are not a contraindication to dental implant therapy; and dental implants can have success and survival rates of up to 100% in patients with RD, such as osteoporosis and RA. However, it is imperative to interpret these results with caution, as most of the studies in this regard had short-term follow-ups or were based on outcomes of case-reports or case-series. Moreover, it is also noteworthy that all patients with RD in whom dental implant therapy yielded fruitful outcomes had "controlled" osteoporosis – that is, they were seeking therapy for their rheumatological disorder. Furthermore, it seems that these patients were actively and regularly maintaining their oral hygiene status, which plays a critical role in the success and survival of dental implants even in patients without an immunocompromised health status (Al Amri et al., 2016). However, the contribution of oral hygiene maintenance toward the overall success and survival of dental implants in patients with RD remained poorly addressed in the studies reviewed.

(a)

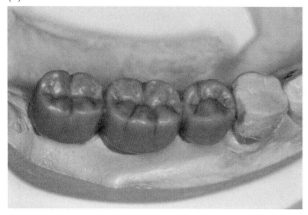

(b)

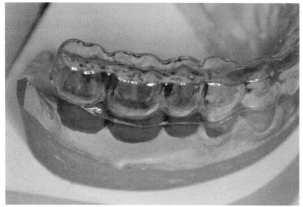

Surgical and Prosthetic Treatment: Dr. Georgios Romanos (Stony Brook, NY, USA)
Dental technician: Axel Calderon (Design Vision, Smithtown, NY, USA)

Figure 17.8 Diagnostic wax up before implant placement (a) and Omnivac® template to be used as radiological, surgical/prosthetic guide (b).

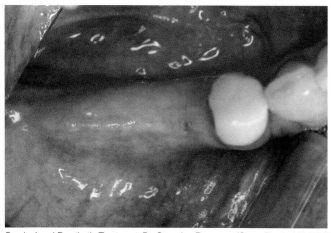

Surgical and Prosthetic Treatment: Dr. Georgios Romanos (Stony Brook, NY, USA)
Dental technician: Axel Calderon (Design Vision, Smithtown, NY, USA)

Figure 17.9 Clinical condition immediately before surgery. The patient suffers with rheumatoid arthritis.

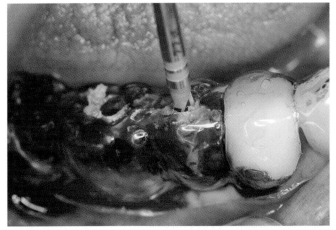

Figure 17.10 Implant positioning using the prosthetic guide.

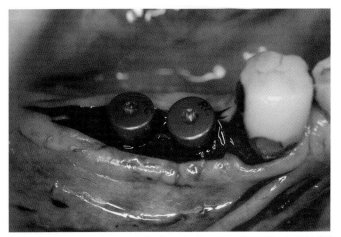

Figure 17.11 Implants placed with regular platform of 4.1mm diameter. (Straumann bone level tapered implants).

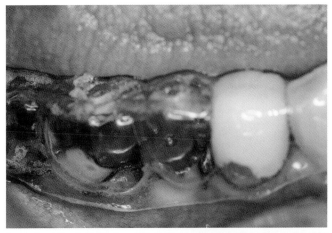

Figure 17.12 Verification of the implant position using the prosthetic guide.

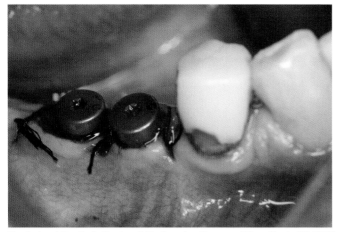

Figure 17.13 Flap sutured in place with silk suturing material (4-0).

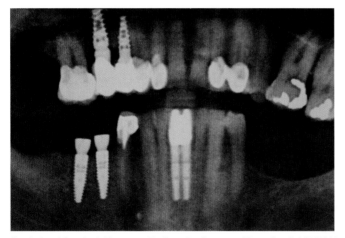

Figure 17.14 Radiographic evaluation immediately after surgery.

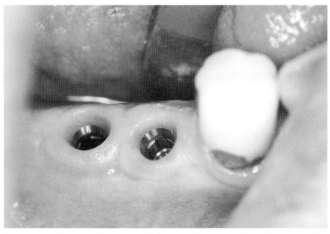

Figure 17.15 Soft peri-implant tissue before delivery of the final restoration.

Conclusion
It seems that dental implants can remain functionally stable in the long term among patients with RD. However, further long-term studies are warranted in this regard. GRADE ACCORDING TO LEVEL OF EVIDENCE: **D**

References

Al Amri, M. D., Kellesarian, S. V., Al-Kheraif, A. A., Malmstrom, H., Javed, F. and Romanos, G. E. 2016. Effect of oral hygiene maintenance on HbA1c levels and peri-implant parameters around immediately-loaded dental implants placed in type-2 diabetic patients: 2 years follow-up. *Clinical Oral Implants Research* 27, pp. 1439–1443. doi:10.1111/clr.12758.

Choi, H. K. 2005. Dietary risk factors for rheumatic diseases. *Current Opinion in Rheumatology* 17, pp. 141–146.

Clarke, A. and Vyse, T. J. 2009. Genetics of rheumatic disease. *Arthritis Research & Therapy* 11, pp. 248. doi:10.1186/ar2781.

Dao, T. T., Anderson, J. D. and Zarb, G. A. 1993. Is osteoporosis a risk factor for osseointegration of dental implants? *The International Journal of Oral & Maxillofacial Implants* 8, pp. 137–144.

Ella, B., Lasserre, J. F., Blanchard, J. P. and Fricain, J. C. 2011. A 4-year follow-up of two complete mandibular implant-supported removable prostheses in a patient with severe rheumatoid polyarthritis: case report. *The International Journal of Oral & Maxillofacial Implants* 26, pp. e19–22.

Giro, G., Chambrone, L., Goldstein, A., Rodrigues, J. A., Zenobio, E., Feres, M., Figueiredo, L. C., Cassoni, A. and Shibli, J. A. 2015. Impact of osteoporosis in dental implants: A systematic review. *World Journal of Orthopology* 6, pp. 311–315. doi:10.5312/wjo.v6.i2.311.

Gremese, E., Tolusso, B., Gigante, M. R. and Ferraccioli, G. 2014. Obesity as a risk and severity factor in rheumatic diseases (autoimmune chronic inflammatory diseases). *Frontiers in Immunolology* 5, pp. 576. doi:10.3389/fimmu.2014.00576.

Holahan, C. M., Koka, S., Kennel, K. A., Weaver, A. L., Assad, D. A., Regennitter, F. J. and Kademani, D. 2008. Effect of osteoporotic status on the survival of titanium dental implants. *International Journal of Oral and Maxillofacial Implants* 23, pp. 905–910.

Kallberg, H., Ding, B., Padyukov, L., Bengtsson, C., Ronnelid, J., Klareskog, L. and Alfredsson, L. 2011. Smoking is a major preventable risk factor for rheumatoid arthritis: estimations of risks after various exposures to cigarette smoke. *Annals of Rheumatic Diseases* 70, pp. 508–511. doi:10.1136/ard.2009.120899.

Krennmair, G., Seemann, R. and Piehslinger, E. 2010. Dental implants in patients with rheumatoid arthritis: clinical outcome and peri-implant findings. *Journal of Clinical Periodontology* 37, pp. 928–936. doi:10.1111/j.1600-051X.2010.01606.x.

Niedermaier, R., Stelzle, F., Riemann, M., Bolz, W., Schuh, P. and Wachtel, H. 2017. Implant-Supported Immediately Loaded Fixed Full-Arch Dentures: Evaluation of Implant Survival Rates in a Case Cohort of up to 7 Years. *Clinical Implant Dentistry and Related Research* 19, pp. 4–19. doi:10.1111/cid.12421.

Pedro, R. E., De Carli, J. P., Linden, M. S., Lima, I. F., Paranhos, L. R., Costa, M. D. and Bos, A. J. 2017. Influence of age on factors associated with peri-implant bone loss after prosthetic rehabilitation over osseointegrated implants. *Journal of Contemporary Dental Practices* 18, pp. 3–10.

Siebert, T., Jurkovic, R., Statelova, D. and Strecha, J. 2015. Immediate implant placement in a patient with osteoporosis undergoing bisphosphonate therapy: 1-year preliminary prospective study. *Journal of Oral Implantology* 41 Spec No, pp. 360–365. doi:10.1563/aaid-joi-d-13-00063.

Tadinada, A., Ortiz, D., Taxel, P., Shafer, D., Rengasamy, K., Pendrys, D. and Freilich, M. 2015. CBCT evaluation of buccal bone regeneration in postmenopausal women with and without osteopenia or osteoporosis undergoing dental implant therapy. *Journal of Prosthetic Dentistry* 114, pp. 498–505. doi:10.1016/j.prosdent.2015.02.015.

Temmerman, A., Rasmusson, L., Kubler, A., Thor, A. and Quirynen, M. 2017. An open, prospective, non-randomized, controlled, multicentre study to evaluate the clinical outcome of implant treatment in women over 60 years of age with osteoporosis/osteopenia: 1-year results. *Clin Oral Implants Res* 28, pp. 95–102. doi:10.1111/clr.12766.

Wagner, F., Schuder, K., Hof, M., Heuberer, S., Seemann, R. and Dvorak, G. 2017. Does osteoporosis influence the marginal peri-implant bone level in female patients? A cross-sectional study in a matched collective. *Clinical Implant Dentistry and Related Research.* doi:10.1111/cid.12493.

Weinlander, M., Krennmair, G. and Piehslinger, E. 2010. Implant prosthodontic rehabilitation of patients with rheumatic disorders: a case series report. *International Journal of Prosthodontics* 23, pp. 22–28.

18

Dental Implants in Patients with Scleroderma

Introduction

Scleroderma (or systemic sclerosis) is a rare autoimmune disease in which hardening and tightening of the skin (Figure 18.1) and connective tissues occurs (Li et al., 2017). Mostly, scleroderma affects only the skin; however, in some cases, it affects other systems such as the vascular system, digestive system, and respiratory tract (Baqir et al., 2017; Gleason et al., 2017). The most common orofacial manifestations of scleroderma are xerostomia, gingival fibrosis, limited mouth opening, widening of the periodontal ligament, and

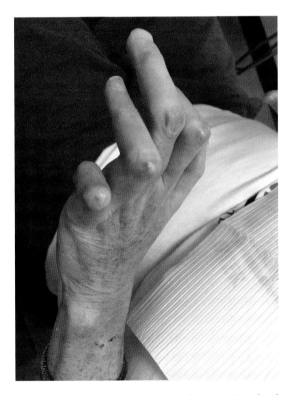

Figure 18.1 Patient with scleroderma demonstrating the characteristic chronic hardening and skin tightening in the fingers.

Evidence-based Implant Dentistry and Systemic Conditions, First Edition.
Fawad Javed and Georgios E. Romanos.
© 2018 John Wiley & Sons, Inc. Published 2018 by John Wiley & Sons, Inc.

trigeminal neuralgia (Baptist, 2016; Hadj Said et al., 2016). Limited mouth opening in these patients may also be associated to esophageal involvement (Vincent et al., 2009).

Results

The literature with respect to the success and survival of dental implants in patients with scleroderma is sparse and the level of available evidence is based on case-reports (Langer et al., 1992; Raviv et al., 1996; Patel et al., 1998; Haas, 2002; Samet et al., 2007; Zigdon et al., 2011; Nam et al., 2012; Baptist, 2016). Some of the case-reports have merely shown that rehabilitation with dental implants is a potent treatment strategy in patients with scleroderma (Langer et al., 1992; Raviv et al., 1996; Haas, 2002). In these studies, the authors emphasized that dental implants should be considered during treatment planning for partially and completely edentulous patients with scleroderma (Langer et al., 1992; Raviv et al., 1996; Haas, 2002). Moreover, the follow-up durations in some of the studies are relatively short (up to three years). A summary of the studies assessing the success and survival of dental implants in patients with scleroderma is shown in Table 18.1.

Conclusion
There is insufficient evidence to determine whether, in the long-term, dental implants can remain functionally stable in patients with scleroderma. Hence, further studies are warranted in this regard.
GRADE ACCORDING TO LEVEL OF EVIDENCE: **D**

Table 18.1 Studies assessing the outcome of dental implant therapy among patients with scleroderma.

Author et al. (Year)	Study design	Age	Gender	Implant location	Follow-up	Outcome
Langer et al. (1992)	Case-report	54 years	Female	Mandible	None	Dental implants can osseointegrate and remain functionally stable in patients with scleroderma.
Raviv et al. (1996)	Case-report	65 years	Female	Mandible	None	Dental implants can osseointegrate and remain functionally stable in patients with scleroderma.
Patel et al. (1998)	Case-report	54 years	Female	Mandible	None	Dental implants can osseointegrate and remain functionally stable in patients with scleroderma.
Haas, S. E. (2002)	Case-report	49 years	Female	Maxilla	None	Dental implants can osseointegrate and remain functionally stable in patients with scleroderma.
Zigdon et al. (2011)	Case-report	45 years	Female	Maxilla and mandible	3 years	All implants were stable at follow-up. Full mouth rehabilitation with dental implants is possible in patients with scleroderma.
Nam et al. (2012)	Case-report	71 years	Female	Maxilla and mandible	None	Full mouth rehabilitation with dental implants is possible in patients with scleroderma.
Baptist (2016)	Case-report	61 years	Female	Posterior maxilla	2 years	All implants were stable at follow-up.

References

Baptist, B. A. 2016. Fixed implant supported rehabilitation of partially edentulous posterior maxilla in a patient with systemic scleroderma: a case report. *Implant Dentistry* 25, pp. 155–159. doi:10.1097/id.0000000000000367.

Baqir, M., Makol, A., Osborn, T. G., Bartholmai, B. J. and Ryu, J. H. 2017. Mycophenolate mofetil for scleroderma-related interstitial lung disease: A real-world experience. *PLoS One* 12, pp. e0177107. doi:10.1371/journal.pone.0177107.

Gleason, J. B., Patel, K. B., Hernandez, F., Hadeh, A., Highland, K. B., Rahaghi, F. and Mehta, J. P. 2017. Pulmonary artery dimensions as a prognosticator of transplant-free survival in scleroderma interstitial lung disease. *Lung*. doi:10.1007/s00408-017-0005-6.

Haas, S. E. 2002. Implant-supported, long-span fixed partial denture for a scleroderma patient: a clinical report. *Journal of Prosthetic Dentistry* 87, pp. 136–139.

Hadj Said, M., Foletti, J. M., Graillon, N., Guyot, L. and Chossegros, C. 2016. Orofacial manifestations of scleroderma. A literature review. *Rev Stomatol Chir Maxillofac Chir Orale* 117, pp. 322–326. doi:10.1016/j.revsto.2016.06.003.

Langer, Y., Cardash, H. S. and Tal, H. 1992. Use of dental implants in the treatment of patients with scleroderma: a clinical report. *Journal of Prosthetic Dentistry* 68, pp. 873–875.

Li, T., Liu, Y. and Xu, H. 2017. Successful treatment of infliximab in a patient with scleroderma: a case report. *Medicine (Baltimore)* 96, pp. e6737. doi:10.1097/md.0000000000006737.

Nam, J., Janakievski, J. and Raigrodski, A. J. 2012. Complete transition from failing restorations to implant-supported fixed prostheses in a patient with scleroderma. *Compendium of Continuing Education in Dentistry* 33, pp. 746–756.

Patel, K., Welfare, R. and Coonar, H. S. 1998. The provision of dental implants and a fixed prosthesis in the treatment of a patient with scleroderma: a clinical report. *Journal of Prosthetic Dentistry* 79, pp. 611–612.

Raviv, E., Harel-Raviv, M., Shatz, P. and Gornitsky, M. 1996. Implant-supported overdenture rehabilitation and progressive systemic sclerosis. *International Journal of Prosthodontics* 9, pp. 440–444.

Samet, N., Tau, S., Findler, M., Susarla, S. M. and Findler, M. 2007. Flexible, removable partial denture for a patient with systemic sclerosis (scleroderma) and microstomia: a clinical report and a three-year follow-up. *General Dentistry* 55, pp. 548–551.

Vincent, C., Agard, C., Barbarot, S., N'Guyen, J. M., Planchon, B., Durant, C., Pistorius, M. A., Dreno, B., Ponge, T., Stalder, J. F., Mercier, J. M. and Hamidou, M. 2009. Orofacial manifestations of systemic sclerosis: a study of 30 consecutive patients. *Rev Med Interne* 30, pp. 5–11. doi:10.1016/j.revmed.2008.06.012.

Zigdon, H., Gutmacher, Z., Teich, S. and Levin, L. 2011. Full-mouth rehabilitation using dental implants in a patient with scleroderma. *Quintessence International* 42, pp. 781–785.

19

Dental Implants in Patients with Sjögren's Syndrome

Introduction

What is Sjögren's Syndrome?

Sjögren's syndrome (SS) is an autoimmune chronic inflammatory disorder characterized by lymphocytic infiltration and destruction of exocrine glands (Korfage et al., 2016; Santosh et al., 2017). Primary SS occurs in the absence of another underlying rheumatic disorder, whereas secondary SS is associated with another underlying rheumatic disease, such as rheumatoid arthritis (RA), systemic lupus erythematosus (SLE) or scleroderma. Classical clinical manifestations of SS are dryness of mucosa of particularly the eyes and oral cavity (Albrecht et al., 2016; Xin et al., 2016). Salivary flow and protein content is also altered among patients with SS, which in turn predisposes these patients to oral diseases such as dental caries, oral *Candida* infections and possibly periodontal disease (Ergun et al., 2010; Katsiougiannis and Wong, 2016; Xin et al., 2016).

Epidemiology of Sjögren's Syndrome

A limited number of studies have investigated the epidemiology of SS; and the incidence and prevalence of SS varies according to the classification criteria used (such as the Copenhagen criteria, the European classification criteria and the International Collaborative Clinical Alliances Cohort) (Patel and Shahane, 2014). Due to selection and misclassification biases, the reported figures are difficult to interpret precisely. The prevalence of primary SS varies between countries and the classification criteria used. In Denmark and Sweden, the prevalence of primary SS has been reported as 0.2%–2.1%, and 2.7%, respectively (Patel and Shahane, 2014); whereas the prevalence of secondary SS has been reported to range between 6.5%–19% (Patel and Shahane, 2014). In the United States, 1 to 2 million individuals have SS; and the reported prevalence ranges between 0.05% and 4.8% (Pillemer et al., 2001).

Figures 19.1 to 19.12 illustrate dental implants in patients with Sjögren's syndrome.

Hypothesis

Since SS is associated with xerostomia and altered salivary function (Albrecht et al., 2016; Katsiougiannis and Wong, 2016), it is hypothesized that SS increases the risk of early implant failure.

Evidence-based Implant Dentistry and Systemic Conditions, First Edition.
Fawad Javed and Georgios E. Romanos.
© 2018 John Wiley & Sons, Inc. Published 2018 by John Wiley & Sons, Inc.

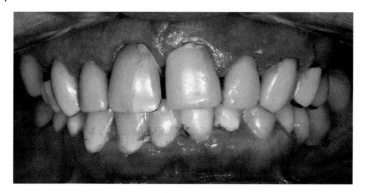

Figure 19.1 Preclinical situation of a patient with type II diabetes. (*Source*: Peron et al., 2017).

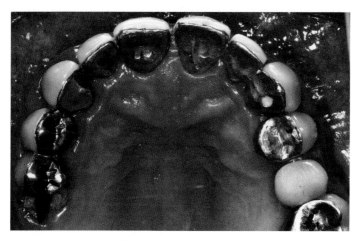

Figure 19.2 Preclinical situation of a patient with Sjogren's Syndrome type II with rheumatoid arthritis.

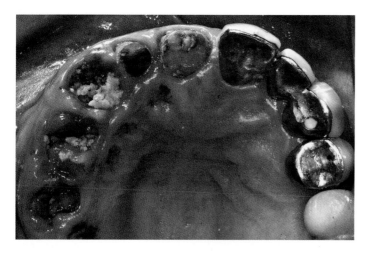

Figure 19.3a Teeth 21-22-23-24-25 with hopeless prognosis.

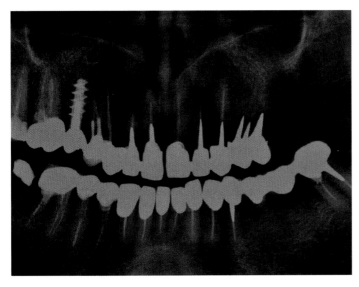

Figure 19.3b Panoramic radiograph before treatment.

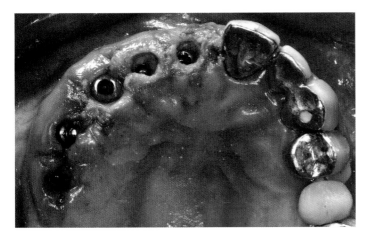

Figure 19.4 Immediate implant placement the day after surgery.

Objective

The aim of this chapter is to review indexed literature to determine whether dental implants can osseointegrate and remain functionally stable in patients with SS.

Materials and Methods

Eligibility Criteria

The following eligibility criteria were entailed: (a) clinical studies and (b) placement and survival of dental implants in adult patients with SS. Literature reviews, letters to the editor, commentaries and articles published in languages other than English were excluded.

Literature Search

PubMed/Medline (National Library of Medicine, Bethesda, Maryland), EMBASE, ISI-Web of Knowledge, SCOPUS and Google-Scholar databases were searched up to February 2018 using the following key words in different combinations: "Sjogren's syndrome," "dental implant," "immunocompromised," "osseointegration," "survival," and "success." Titles and abstracts of studies that fulfilled the eligibility criteria were screened and checked for agreement. Full texts of studies judged by title and abstract to be relevant were read and assessed

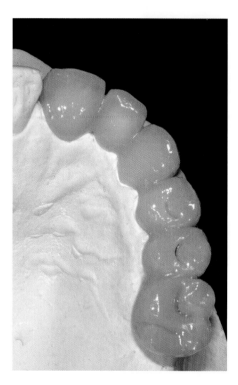

Figure 19.5 Provisional restoration.

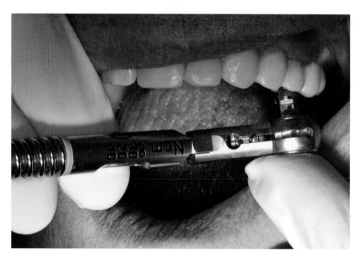

Figure 19.6a Immediate loading with screw-retained provisional restoration (torque: 30 Ncm).

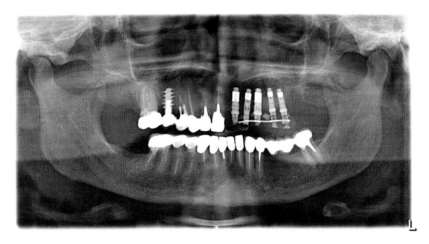

Figure 19.6b Radiograph taken after surgery with immediate provisional restoration.

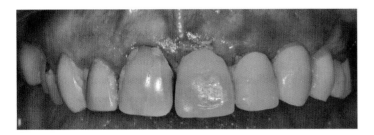

Figure 19.7 Immediate provisional restoration in place the day after surgery.

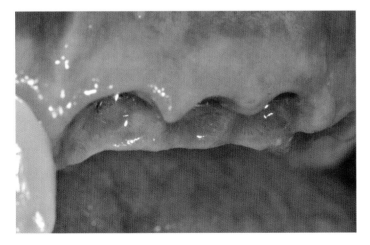

Figure 19.8 Excellent healing of soft tissues after removal of temporary restoration after 4 months.

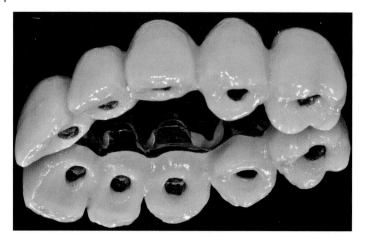

Figure 19.9 Final restoration in metal/ceramic.

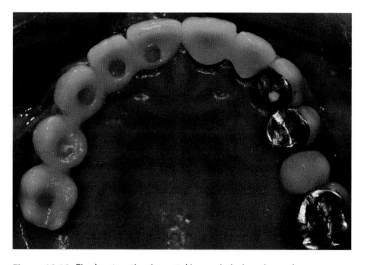

Figure 19.10 Final restoration in metal/ceramic (mirror image).

in accordance with the eligibility criteria (as stated above). In addition, hand searching of the reference lists of potentially relevant original and review studies was also performed and checked for agreement via discussion.

Results

In total, seven studies (Payne et al., 1997; Isidor et al., 1999; Binon, 2005; Spinato et al., 2010; Albrecht et al., 2016; Korfage et al., 2016; Peron et al., 2017) were identified and processed for data extraction. Two studies were case-series (Payne et al., 1997; Isidor et al., 1999), two were case-reports (Binon, 2005; Spinato et al., 2010), and two (Albrecht et al., 2016; Korfage et al., 2016) had a cohort design. In these studies, the participants were mostly females, and dental implants were placed in both jaws. The follow-up duration ranged between 1 and 13 years.

Figure 19.11 a and b Smileline of the patient.

(a)

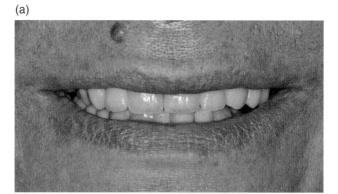

(b)

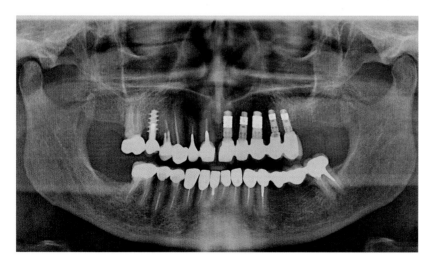

Figure 19.12 Radiographic view 3 years after treatment.

The implant survival rate was reported in four studies (Payne et al., 1997; Binon, 2005; Spinato et al., 2010; Korfage et al., 2016), which ranged between 97% and 100%. In the study by Peron et al. (2017), Tantalum-based dental implants placed in the edentulous maxilla of a female patient remained functionally stable up to 30 months of follow-up. These results are summarized in Table 19.1.

Table 19.1 Studies assessing the outcome of dental implant therapy among patients with Sjögren's syndrome.

Authors et al. (Year)	Study design	Patient/s with SS (n)	SS patient/s with dental implants	Age/Mean age of patients with SS	Duration of SS	Number of implants failed/placed (n)	Jaw location	Duration of follow-up	Implant survival rate	Outcome
Payne et al. (1997)	Case-series	3	3	Patient 1: 38 years Patient 2: 38 years Patient 3: 40 years	Patient 1: 16 years Patient 2: 15 years Patient 3: NA	Patient 1: 0/6 Patient 2: 0/6 Patient 3: 0/8	Patient 1: Maxilla and mandible Patient 2: Maxilla and mandible Patient 3: Maxilla and mandible	Patient 1: 8 years* Patient 2: 1 year* Patient 3: 1 year*	Patient 1: 100% Patient 2: 100% Patient 3: 100%	Dental implants can remain functionally stable in patients with SS.
Isidor et al. (1999)	Case-series	8	8	NA (range: 53–70 years)	NA	7/54	Maxilla and mandible	4 years	NA	Dental implants remained functionally stable in the patient up to follow-up.
Binon et al. (2005)	Case-report	1	1	67 years	NA	0/6	Mandible	13 years*	100%	Dental implants can remain functionally stable in patients with SS.
Spinato et al. (2010)	Case-report	1	1	62 years	7 years	0	Mandible	1 year	100%	Dental implants remained functionally stable in the patient up to follow-up.
Albrecht et al. (2016)	Observational cohort	230 females	32 females	64.5 years	NA	5/104	NA	4.9 years*	NA	Dental implants can remain functionally stable in patients with SS.
Korfage et al. (2016)	Retrospective cohort	50	50	67 ± 8 years	9 years	4/142	Edentulous mandible	3.8 years*	97%	Dental implants can remain functionally stable in patients with SS.
Peron et al. (2017)	Case-report	1	1	62 years	6 years	0/5	Maxilla	2.5 years	100%	Dental implants remained functionally stable in the patient up to follow-up.

*The implants had been in function since this time duration
NA: Not available

Discussion

The literature search showed that there are only a limited number of studies (Payne et al., 1997; Isidor et al., 1999; Binon, 2005; Spinato et al., 2010; Albrecht et al., 2016; Korfage et al., 2016; Peron et al., 2017) that have assessed the success/survival of dental implants in patients with SS. Most of the studies were either case-reports (Isidor et al., 1999; Binon, 2005; Spinato et al., 2010) or case-series (Payne et al., 1997). In addition, the two cohort (Albrecht et al., 2016; Korfage et al., 2016) studies that assessed the survival of dental implants in patients with SS had follow-up durations of approximately four and five years. However, from the literature reviewed, it seems that dental implants can remain functionally stable in patients with SS. Further prospective and retrospective studies on patients with SS with a larger patient population and long-term follow-up (>5 years) are needed to assess the survival of dental implants in patients with SS.

Conclusion
There is insufficient evidence to determine whether dental implants can remain functionally stable in the long-term among patients with SS. Hence, further studies are warranted in this regard.
GRADE ACCORDING TO LEVEL OF EVIDENCE: **D**

References

Albrecht, K., Callhoff, J., Westhoff, G., Dietrich, T., Dorner, T. and Zink, A. 2016. The prevalence of dental implants and related factors in patients with Sjogren syndrome: Results from a cohort study. *Journal of Rheumatology* 43, pp. 1380–1385. doi:10.3899/jrheum.151167.

Binon, P. P. 2005. Thirteen-year follow-up of a mandibular implant-supported fixed complete denture in a patient with Sjogren's syndrome: a clinical report. *Journal of Prosthetic Dentistry* 94, pp. 409–413. doi:10.1016/j.prosdent.2005.09.010.

Ergun, S., Cekici, A., Topcuoglu, N., Migliari, D. A., Kulekci, G., Tanyeri, H. and Isik, G. 2010. Oral status and Candida colonization in patients with Sjogren's syndrome. *Medicina Oral Patologia Oral y Cirugia Bucal* 15, pp. e310–315.

Isidor, F., Brondum, K., Hansen, H. J., Jensen, J. and Sindet-Pedersen, S. 1999. Outcome of treatment with implant-retained dental prostheses in patients with Sjogren syndrome. *The International Journal of Oral & Maxillofacial Implants* 14, pp. 736–743.

Katsiougiannis, S. and Wong, D. T. 2016. The proteomics of saliva in sjogren's syndrome. *Rheumatic Diseases Clinics of North America* 42, pp. 449–456. doi:10.1016/j.rdc.2016.03.004.

Korfage, A., Raghoebar, G. M., Arends, S., Meiners, P. M., Visser, A., Kroese, F. G., Bootsma, H. and Vissink, A. 2016. Dental implants in patients with Sjogren's syndrome. *Clinical Implant Dentistry and Related Research* 18, pp. 937–945. doi:10.1111/cid.12376.

Patel, R. and Shahane, A. 2014. The epidemiology of Sjogren's syndrome. *Clinical Epidemiology* 6, pp. 247–255. doi:10.2147/clep.s47399.

Payne, A. G., Lownie, J. F. and Van Der Linden, W. J. 1997. Implant-supported prostheses in patients with Sjogren's syndrome: a clinical report on three patients. *The International Journal of Oral & Maxillofacial Implants* 12, pp. 679–685.

Peron, C., Javed, F. and Romanos, G. E. 2017. Immediate loading of tantalum-based implants in fresh extraction sockets in patient with Sjogren syndrome: A case report and literature review. *Implant Dentistry* 26(4), pp. 634–638. doi:10.1097/id.0000000000000594.

Pillemer, S. R., Matteson, E. L., Jacobsson, L. T., Martens, P. B., Melton, L. J., 3rd, O'Fallon, W. M. and Fox, P. C. 2001. Incidence of physician-diagnosed primary Sjogren syndrome in residents of Olmsted County, Minnesota. *Mayo Clinic Proceedings* 76, pp. 593–599. doi:10.4065/76.6.593.

Santosh, K., Dhir, V., Singh, S., Sood, A., Gupta, A., Sharma, A. and Sharma, S. 2017. Prevalence of secondary Sjogren's syndrome in Indian patients with rheumatoid arthritis: a single-center study. *International Journal of Rheumatic Diseases* 20(7), 870–874. doi:10.1111/1756-185x.13017.

Spinato, S., Soardi, C. M. and Zane, A. M. 2010. A mandibular implant-supported fixed complete dental prosthesis in a patient with Sjogren syndrome: case report. *Implant Dentistry* 19, pp. 178–183. doi:10.1097/ID.0b013e3181dbe081.

Xin, W., Leung, K. C., Lo, E. C., Mok, M. Y. and Leung, M. H. 2016. A randomized, double-blind, placebo-controlled clinical trial of fluoride varnish in preventing dental caries of Sjogren's syndrome patients. *BMC Oral Health* 16, pp. 102. doi:10.1186/s12903-016-0296-7.

20

Dental Implants in Patients Who Habitually Use Smokeless Tobacco Products

Types of Smokeless Tobacco

Several varieties of smokeless tobacco (ST) products are commercially available despite the imposition of a ban on the manufacturing and sale of such products by some countries. The most commonly used ST product is snuff, which may be either moist or dry. Moist snuff contains finely ground tobacco that is available either in loose form or in small rectangular pouches. The pouch or ground tobacco is usually placed in the buccal mucosa of the mandibular premolar region (Figure 20.1a). *Gutka* and betel-quid (BQ) are other forms of smokeless tobacco predominantly consumed in South Asia. However, global export has made this form of ST product available to several migrant communities living in Europe, Australia, and North America (Changrani et al., 2006; Benowitz et al., 2012; Banerjee et al., 2014). Gutka is a blend of powdered tobacco, slaked lime (aqueous calcium hydroxide paste), finely ground areca nut, and artificial fragrances (Figure 20.1b). The BQ is a mixture of areca nut, artificial sweeteners and fragrances, slaked lime, and sometimes powdered tobacco wrapped in *piper betle* leaf (Figure 20.1c) (Javed et al., 2008; Javed et al., 2010; Javed et al., 2014). *Gutka* and BQ are initially placed in the mouth between the upper and lower posterior teeth and gently chewed and sucked sporadically. The contents of both forms of ST are held against the buccal vestibule over prolonged durations and continued to be gentle chewed and sucked. The contents may either be spat out or swallowed when desired.

Effect of Habitual Smokeless Tobacco Consumption on Oral Health

Several studies have reported that oral health status is compromised in individuals habitually using ST products as compared to controls (individuals not using tobacco in any form) (Wickholm et al., 2004; Javed et al., 2008; Javed et al., 2010; Hugoson and Rolandsson, 2011; Javed et al., 2013; Javed et al., 2014; Mallery et al., 2014). Clinical and radiographic results have reported worse periodontal status (in terms of increased plaque index, bleeding on probing, probing pocket depth, and marginal bone loss) among habitual ST users as compared to controls (Wickholm et al., 2004; Javed et al., 2008; Javed et al., 2010; Hugoson and Rolandsson, 2011; Javed et al., 2013; Javed et al., 2014). Moreover, an increased prevalence of oral precancer and cancer has been reported in individuals using ST products as compared to controls (Javed et al., 2010; Chandra and Govindraju, 2012;

Evidence-based Implant Dentistry and Systemic Conditions, First Edition.
Fawad Javed and Georgios E. Romanos.
© 2018 John Wiley & Sons, Inc. Published 2018 by John Wiley & Sons, Inc.

(a)   (b)   (c)

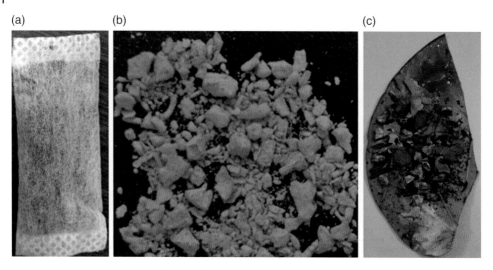

Figure 20.1 Forms of commercially available smokeless tobacco products (a) snuff; (b) gutka, and (c) betel-quid.

Hirsch et al., 2012; Sujatha et al., 2012; Kavarodi et al., 2014; Sridharan, 2014). The aim of this chapter was to review indexed literature to determine whether dental implants can osseointegrate and remain functionally stable in habitual ST product users.

Smokeless Tobacco Products and Dental Implants

Following an exhaustive search of indexed literature, we found no studies that assessed the osseointegration and survival of dental implants in habitual ST product users (Table 20.1). However, based on our current knowledge about the hazardous effects of the components of ST products on oral and periodontal health status, we are tempted to speculate that habitual ST chewing negatively influences the osseointegration and long-term survival of dental implants. It is known that areca nut (a major component in ST products) contains alkaloids (such as arecoline), which induce oxidative stress in oral keratinocytes and cell death (Thangjam and Kondaiah, 2009). In addition, in-vitro results have shown that arecoline is cytotoxic to human gingival fibroblasts; and frequent and

Table 20.1 Characteristics and outcome of the study that assessed osseointegration and survival of dental implants in habitual smokeless tobacco product users.

Authors et al. (Year)	Mean age (Range)	Gender	Form of smokeless tobacco used	Duration of habit	Daily frequency of habit	Number of implants placed	Jaw location	Follow-up	Outcome

No Studies in Indexed Literature

long-term exposure to arecoline could impair the function of gingival fibroblasts (Chang et al., 1999). Areca-nut chewing has also been associated with the etiology of systemic disorders such as metabolic syndrome, which is also a significant risk factor for periodontal bone loss (Nesbitt et al., 2010; Javed et al., 2012; Jin et al., 2014).

Nicotine from powdered tobacco (an essential component of ST products) has been shown to enhance the effects of the local components of periodontal disease in a non-dose-dependent manner (Nociti et al., 2000). Results from a study on rats showed that nicotine influences alveolar bone changes by enhancing bone loss (Nogueira-Filho et al., 2004). Furthermore, other components of ST products (such as slaked lime) alkaline conditions in the oral cavity thereby favoring the production of reactive oxygen species (ROS), which play a role in augmenting oral mucosal inflammation and carcinogenesis (Nair et al., 1990).

Conclusion

There are no studies in indexed literature that have assessed whether dental implants can osseointegrate and remain functionally stable in habitual ST product users. Hence, further studies are warranted in this regard.

GRADE ACCORDING TO LEVEL OF EVIDENCE: **D**

References

Banerjee, S. C., Ostroff, J. S., Bari, S., D'Agostino, T. A., Khera, M., Acharya, S. and Gany, F. (2014). Gutka and Tambaku Paan use among South Asian immigrants: a focus group study. *Journal of Immigrant and Minority Health* 16, pp. 531–539. doi:10.1007/s10903-013-9826-4.

Benowitz, N. L., Renner, C. C., Lanier, A. P., Tyndale, R. F., Hatsukami, D. K., Lindgren, B., Stepanov, I., Watson, C. H., Sosnoff, C. S. and Jacob, P., III (2012). Exposure to nicotine and carcinogens among Southwestern Alaskan Native cigarette smokers and smokeless tobacco users. *Cancer Epidemiology Biomarkers Prev* 21, pp. 934–942. doi:10.1158/1055-9965.epi-11-1178.

Chandra, P. and Govindraju, P. (2012). Prevalence of oral mucosal lesions among tobacco users. *Oral Health Preventative Dentistry* 10, pp. 149–153.

Chang, Y. C., Tai, K. W., Lii, C. K., Chou, L. S. and Chou, M. Y. (1999). Cytopathologic effects of arecoline on human gingival fibroblasts in vitro. *Clinical Oral Investigations* 3, pp. 25–29.

Changrani, J., Gany, F. M., Cruz, G., Kerr, R. and Katz, R. (2006). Paan and Gutka Use in the United States: A Pilot Study in Bangladeshi and Indian-Gujarati Immigrants in New York City. *Journal of Immigrant & Refugee Studies* 4, pp. 99–110. doi:10.1300/J500v04n01_07.

Hirsch, J. M., Wallstrom, M., Carlsson, A. P. and Sand, L. (2012). Oral cancer in Swedish snuff dippers. *Anticancer Research* 32, pp. 3327–3330.

Hugoson, A. and Rolandsson, M. (2011). Periodontal disease in relation to smoking and the use of Swedish snus: epidemiological studies covering 20 years (1983–2003). *Journal of Clinical Periodontology* 38, pp. 809–816.

Javed, F., Al-Hezaimi, K. and Warnakulasuriya, S. (2012). Areca-nut chewing habit is a significant risk factor for metabolic syndrome: a systematic review. *Journal of Nutrition Health and Aging* 16, pp. 445–448.

Javed, F., Altamash, M., Klinge, B. & Engstrom, P. E. (2008) Periodontal conditions and oral symptoms in gutka-chewers with and without type 2 diabetes. *Acta Odontologica Scandinavica* 66, pp. 268–273. doi:10.1080/00016350802286725.

Javed, F., Chotai, M., Mehmood, A. and Almas, K. (2010). Oral mucosal disorders associated with habitual gutka usage: a review. *Oral Surgery, Oral Medicine, Oral Pathology, Oral Radiology, and Endodontology* 109, pp. 857–864. doi:10.1016/j.tripleo.2009.12.038.

Javed, F., Tenenbaum, H. C., Nogueira-Filho, G., Nooh, N., Taiyeb Ali, T. B., Samaranayake, L. P. and Al-Hezaimi, K. (2014). Oral Candida carriage and species prevalence amongst habitual gutka-chewers and non-chewers. *International Wound Journal* 11, pp. 79–84. doi:10.1111/j.1742-481X.2012.01070.x.

Javed, F., Tenenbaum, H. C., Nogueira-Filho, G., Qayyum, F., Correa, F. O., Al-Hezaimi, K. and Samaranayake, L. P. (2013). Severity of periodontal disease in individuals chewing betel quid with and without tobacco. *American Journal of Medical Science* 346, pp. 273–278. doi:10.1097/MAJ.0b013e31827333fb.

Jin, J., Machado, E. R., Yu, H., Zhang, X., Lu, Z., Li, Y., Lopes-Virella, M. F., Kirkwood, K. L. & Huang, Y. (2014). Simvastatin inhibits LPS-induced alveolar bone loss during metabolic syndrome. *Journal of Dental Research* 93, pp. 294–299. doi:10.1177/0022034513516980.

Kavarodi, A. M., Thomas, M. and Kannampilly, J. (2014). Prevalence of oral pre-malignant lesions and its risk factors in an Indian subcontinent low income migrant group in Qatar. *Asian Pacific Journal of Cancer Prevention* 15, pp. 4325–4329.

Mallery, S. R., Tong, M., Michaels, G. C., Kiyani, A. R. and Hecht, S. S. (2014). Clinical and biochemical studies support smokeless tobacco's carcinogenic potential in the human oral cavity. *Cancer Prevention Research (Phila)* 7, pp. 23–32. doi:10.1158/1940-6207.capr-13-0262.

Nair, U. J., Friesen, M., Richard, I., MacLennan, R., Thomas, S. and Bartsch, H. (1990). Effect of lime composition on the formation of reactive oxygen species from areca nut extract in vitro. *Carcinogenesis* 11, pp. 2145–2148.

Nesbitt, M. J., Reynolds, M. A., Shiau, H., Choe, K., Simonsick, E. M. and Ferrucci, L. (2010). Association of periodontitis and metabolic syndrome in the Baltimore Longitudinal Study of Aging. *Aging Clinical and Experimental Research* 22, pp. 238–242.

Nociti, F. H., Jr., Nogueira-Filho, G. R., Primo, M. T., Machado, M. A., Tramontina, V. A., Barros, S. P. and Sallum, E. A. (2000). The influence of nicotine on the bone loss rate in ligature-induced periodontitis. A histometric study in rats. *Journal of Periodontology* 71, pp. 1460–1464. doi:10.1902/jop.2000.71.9.1460.

Nogueira-Filho, G. R., Froes Neto, E. B., Casati, M. Z., Reis, S. R., Tunes, R. S., Tunes, U. R., Sallum, E. A., Nociti, F. H., Jr. and Sallum, A. W. (2004). Nicotine effects on alveolar bone changes induced by occlusal trauma: a histometric study in rats. *Journal of Periodontology* 75, pp. 348–352. doi:10.1902/jop.2004.75.3.348.

Sridharan, G. (2014). Epidemiology, control and prevention of tobacco induced oral mucosal lesions in India. *Indian Journal of Cancer* 51, pp. 80–85.

Sujatha, D., Hebbar, P. B. and Pai, A. (2012). Prevalence and correlation of oral lesions among tobacco smokers, tobacco chewers, areca nut and alcohol users. *Asian Pacific Journal of Cancer Prevention* 13, pp. 1633–1637.

Thangjam, G. S. and Kondaiah, P. (2009). Regulation of oxidative-stress responsive genes by arecoline in human keratinocytes. *Journal of Periodontal Research* 44, pp. 673–682. doi:10.1111/j.1600-0765.2008.01176.x.

Wickholm, S., Soder, P. O., Galanti, M. R., Soder, B. and Klinge, B. (2004). Periodontal disease in a group of Swedish adult snuff and cigarette users. *Acta Odontologica Scandinavica* 62, pp. 333–338.

21

Dental Implants in Patients who Habitually Smoke Tobacco

Smoking: A Classical Risk Factor of Peri-Implant Diseases

Dental implants can demonstrate success and survival rates of up to 100% (Romanos et al., 2014; Calvo-Guirado et al., 2015; Aunmeungtong et al., 2016); however, occurrence of complications, such as peri-implant diseases (peri-implant mucositis and peri-implantitis) cannot be disregarded (Romanos et al., 2015). A significant risk factor of peri-implant diseases is habitual use of tobacco products (Javed et al., 2009; Saaby et al., 2016).

It has been reported that tobacco smoke contains over 4,000 potential toxins, of which, nicotine is considered as one of the most hazardous and addictive (Hoffmann et al., 1997). In a recent retrospective clinical study, Chrcanovic et al. (2016) investigated the local risk factors associated with dental implant failure among 2,670 participants who had received 10,096 implants. The results were based on univariate and multivariate logistic regression models and showed that tobacco smoking is a statistically significant predictor of dental implant failure (Chrcanovic et al., 2016). Similarly, result from a systematic review and meta-analysis also showed that the rates of implant failure, postoperative infections, and peri-implant crestal bone loss are statistically significantly higher in smokers compared with nonsmokers (Keenan and Veitz-Keenan, 2016). Furthermore, it has also been reported that Type IV bone (that exhibits a poor cortical thickness, low trabecular density, and poor medullary strength) is more often seen among smokers compared with nonsmokers (Bain and Moy, 1993).

How Does Nicotine Affect Osseointegration?

A limited number of animal studies have assessed the impact of nicotine on osseointegration (Stefani et al., 2002; Cesar-Neto et al., 2003; Balatsouka et al., 2005a; Balatsouka et al., 2005b; Gotfredsen et al., 2009; Berley et al., 2010; Soares et al., 2010; Yamano et al., 2010). In the studies by Berley et al. (2010) and Yamano et al. (2010), there was a statistically significant decrease in bone-to-implant contacts among rats exposed to nicotine at four-week follow-ups compared with unexposed rats. Results by Soares et al. (2010) showed that bone volume (BV) around implants was significantly lower in rats that received subcutaneous injections of nicotine than control rats.

In contrast, some studies (Stefani et al., 2002; Cesar-Neto et al., 2003; Balatsouka et al., 2005a; Balatsouka et al., 2005b; Gotfredsen et al., 2009) have reported no statistically significant difference in bone-to-implant contacts between in animals with or without nicotine

Evidence-based Implant Dentistry and Systemic Conditions, First Edition.
Fawad Javed and Georgios E. Romanos.
© 2018 John Wiley & Sons, Inc. Published 2018 by John Wiley & Sons, Inc.

administration. However, it is important to interpret these results with caution, as nicotine was administered to the animals subcutaneously in these studies (Stefani et al., 2002; Cesar-Neto et al., 2003; Balatsouka et al., 2005a; Balatsouka et al., 2005b; Gotfredsen et al., 2009). It has been reported that drug (nicotine) absorption is faster through the inhanation route as compared to subcutaneous drug administration (Romich, 2005). Therefore, it is likely that the subcutaneous injections of nicotine was unable to demonstrate the true effects on osseointegration in these studies (Stefani et al., 2002; Cesar-Neto et al., 2003; Balatsouka et al., 2005a; Balatsouka et al., 2005b; Gotfredsen et al., 2009) due to its slow absorption in the systemic circulation.

Success and Survival of Dental Implants in Smokers

Cigarette Smoking

A classical risk factor for peri-implant diseases and implant failure is cigarette smoking (Bain et al., 1993; Wallace, 2000; Vervaeke et al., 2012; Twito and Sade, 2014; Romanos et al., 2015; Sun et al., 2016). Levin et al. (2008) reported that peri-implant mean bone loss (MBL) is statistically significantly higher in cigarette smokers compared with ex-smokers and non-smokers. One explanation in this regard is that nicotine increases the production of inflammatory cytokines (such as interleukin [IL]-6 and tumor necrosis factor-alpha) by osteoblasts (Rosa et al., 2008). However, controversial results have also been reported previously.

Removable implant-supported restorations are recommended in heavy smokers (Figures 21.1 to 21.10). Advanced surgical protocols, such as extensive flap elevations, bone grafting, and immediate implant placement in fresh extraction sockets may be associated with mechanically stable implants but with compromised esthetics (Figures 21.11 to 21.18).

In a study by Romanos et al. (2013), platform-switched implants were placed in smokers (individuals who smoked at least 20 cigarettes daily for over 10 years) and nonsmoking

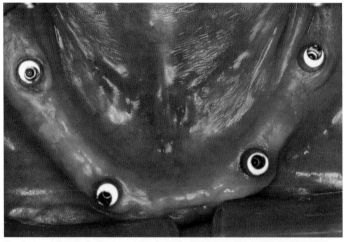

Surgical and Prosthetic Treatment: Dr. Georgios Romanos (Stony Brook, NY, USA)
Dental technician: Axel Calderon (Design Vision, Smithtown, NY, USA)

Figure 21.1 Intraoral condition of a heavy smoker with telescopic implant-supported restoration.

(a)

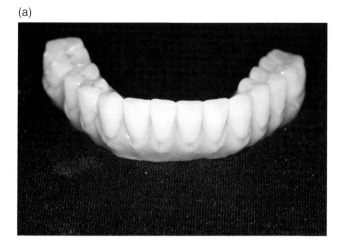

(b)

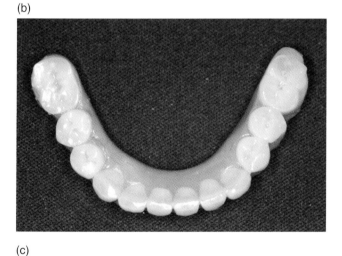

(c)

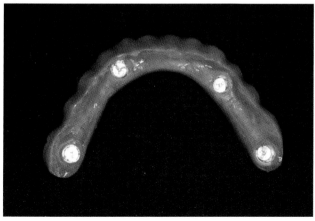

Surgical and Prosthetic Treatment: Dr. Georgios Romanos (Stony Brook, NY, USA)
Dental technician: Axel Calderon (Design Vision, Smithtown, NY, USA)

Figures 21.2a–c Telescopic implant-supported bridge on SynCone abutments (Dentsply-Sirona) presenting excellent esthetic result (a) in occlusal view; (b) base of the prosthesis; (c) allowing high plaque control in heavy smoker.

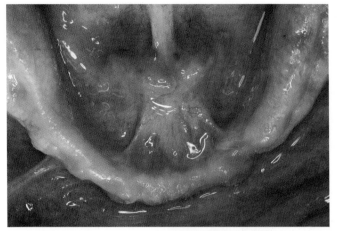

Surgical Treatment: Dr. Georgios Romanos (Stony Brook, NY, USA)
Prosthetic Treatment: Dr. Rafael Delgado-Ruiz (Stony Brook, NY, USA)

Figure 21.3 Preoperative clinical condition of the mandible of a heavy smoker.

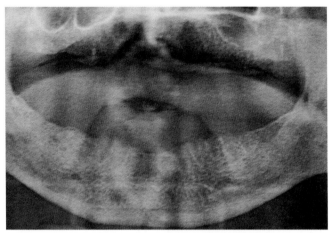

Surgical Treatment: Dr. Georgios Romanos (Stony Brook, NY, USA)
Prosthetic Treatment: Dr. Rafael Delgado-Ruiz (Stony Brook, NY, USA)

Figure 21.4 Radiographic condition presenting very good height in the mandible.

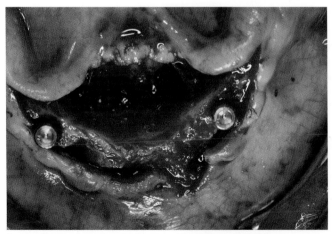

Surgical Treatment: Dr. Georgios Romanos (Stony Brook, NY, USA)
Prosthetic Treatment: Dr. Rafael Delgado-Ruiz (Stony Brook, NY, USA)

Figure 21.5 Implants with narrow diameter (Zest) were placed to restore the patient with an implant-supported overdenture.

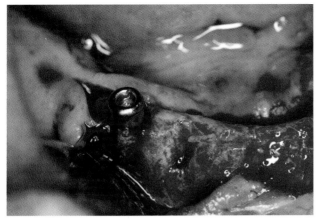

Surgical Treatment: Dr. Georgios Romanos (Stony Brook, NY, USA)
Prosthetic Treatment: Dr. Rafael Delgado-Ruiz (Stony Brook, NY, USA)

Figure 21.6 Implants housed by bone at the right side.

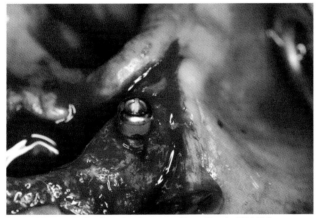

Surgical Treatment: Dr. Georgios Romanos (Stony Brook, NY, USA)
Prosthetic Treatment: Dr. Rafael Delgado-Ruiz (Stony Brook, NY, USA)

Figure 21.7 Implants housed by bone at the left side.

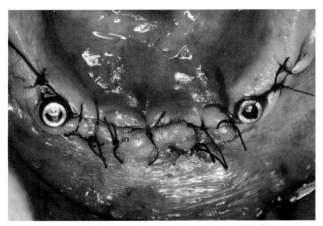

Surgical Treatment: Dr. Georgios Romanos (Stony Brook, NY, USA)
Prosthetic Treatment: Dr. Rafael Delgado-Ruiz (Stony Brook, NY, USA)

Figure 21.8 Surgical site after flap closure.

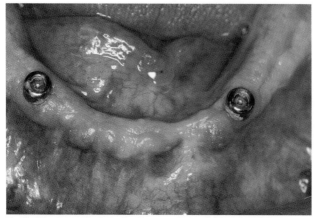

Surgical Treatment: Dr. Georgios Romanos (Stony Brook, NY, USA)
Prosthetic Treatment: Dr. Rafael Delgado-Ruiz (Stony Brook, NY, USA)

Figure 21.9 Implants after 6 months of loading.

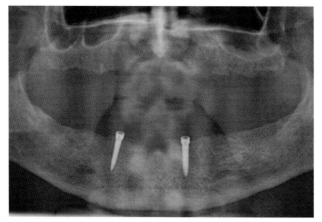

Surgical Treatment: Dr. Georgios Romanos (Stony Brook, NY, USA)
Prosthetic Treatment: Dr. Rafael Delgado-Ruiz (Stony Brook, NY, USA)

Figure 21.10 Radiographic demonstration of the implants 6 months after loading.

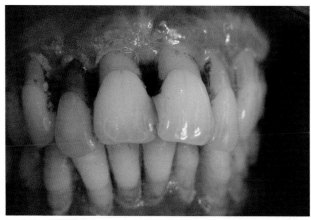

Surgical and Prosthetic Treatment: Dr. Georgios Romanos (Stony Brook, NY, USA)
Dental technician: Marion Biaesch (Frankfurt, Germany)

Figure 21.11 Clinical demonstration of the hopeless dentition in a heavy smoker due to severe periodontitis. (*Source:* Romanos, 2012. Reproduced with permission of Quintessence).

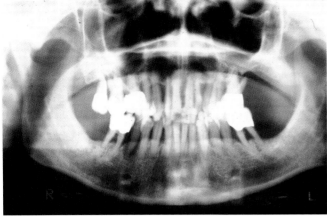

Surgical and Prosthetic Treatment: Dr. Georgios Romanos (Stony Brook, NY, USA)
Dental technician: Marion Biaesch (Frankfurt, Germany)

Figure 21.12 Radiological demonstration of the hopeless dentition in a heavy smoker. (*Source:* Romanos, 2012. Reproduced with permission of Quintessence).

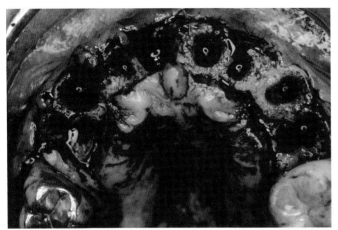

Surgical and Prosthetic Treatment: Dr. Georgios Romanos (Stony Brook, NY, USA)
Dental technician: Marion Biaesch (Frankfurt, Germany)

Figure 21.13 Tooth extraction in the maxilla prepared for immediate implant placement. (*Source:* Romanos, 2012. Reproduced with permission of Quintessence).

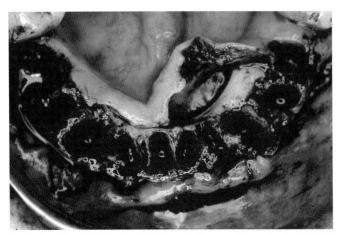

Surgical and Prosthetic Treatment: Dr. Georgios Romanos (Stony Brook, NY, USA)
Dental technician: Marion Biaesch (Frankfurt, Germany)

Figure 21.14 Tooth extraction in the mandible immediately before immediate implant placement. (*Source:* Romanos, 2012. Reproduced with permission of Quintessence).

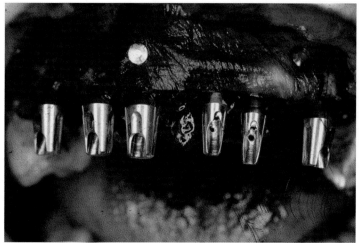

Surgical and Prosthetic Treatment: Dr. Georgios Romanos (Stony Brook, NY, USA)
Dental technician: Marion Biaesch (Frankfurt, Germany)

Figure 21.15 Implant placement in the maxillary fresh extraction socket in conjunction with bone grafting before immediate loading with a fixed prosthesis. (*Source:* Romanos, 2012. Reproduced with permission of Quintessence).

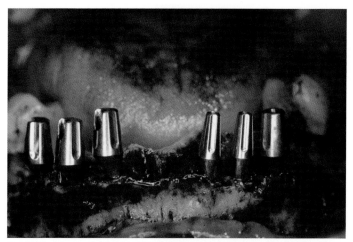

Surgical and Prosthetic Treatment: Dr. Georgios Romanos (Stony Brook, NY, USA)
Dental technician: Marion Biaesch (Frankfurt, Germany)

Figure 21.16 Implant placement in the mandibular fresh extraction socket in conjunction with bone grafting before immediate loading with a fixed prosthesis. (*Source:* Romanos, 2012. Reproduced with permission of Quintessence).

individuals using the same treatment protocol. All implants were immediately loaded and the follow-up periods in smokers and nonsmokers were approximately 5 and 9 years, respectively. At follow-up, implant survival rates were 97% and 99% among smokers and nonsmokers, respectively (Romanos et al., 2013). The study concluded that long-term clinical outcomes for immediately loaded platform-shifted implants placed in smokers and nonsmokers are comparable when the abutments are placed at the day of surgery and never removed (Romanos et al., 2013) (Table 21.1; Figures 21.19 and 21.20).

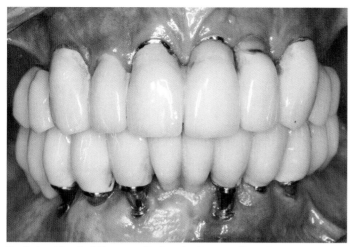

Surgical and Prosthetic Treatment: Dr. Georgios Romanos (Stony Brook, NY, USA)
Dental technician: Marion Biaesch (Frankfurt, Germany)

Figure 21.17 Clinical condition after immediate implant placement and loading in a heavy smoker due to the increased diameter of implants (4.5 mm) used at the day of surgery. The implants were placed immediate after tooth extraction. The clinical photograph was taken 17 years after treatment.

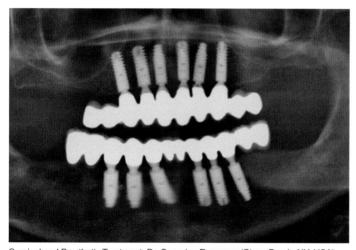

Surgical and Prosthetic Treatment: Dr. Georgios Romanos (Stony Brook, NY, USA)
Dental technician: Marion Biaesch (Frankfurt, Germany)

Figure 21.18 Radiological demonstration of the final outcome 17 years after surgery in a heavy smoker.

Waterpipe Smoking

Waterpipe (synonyms: hookah, hubble bubble, narghile, and sheesha) is a type of tobacco smoking in which charcoal-heated air passes through a perforated aluminium foil and across powdered tobacco to become smoke, which bubbles through water before being inhaled. Waterpipe smoking (WS) is a cultural norm in many countries such as Bahrain, Egypt, Israel, Kuwait, Qatar, Saudi Arabia, and the United Arab Emirates (Natto, 2005; Moh'd Al-Mulla et al., 2008; Borgan et al., 2014; Almutairi, 2015; Jawad et al., 2015;

Table 21.1 Studies assessing the effect of cigarette smoking on the success and survival of dental implants.

Authors et al. (Year)	Study design	Participants	Follow-up	Relationship between cigarette smoking and implant failure	Were the outcomes comparable to nonsmokers?
Bain and Moy (1993)	Cohort	44 smokers	6 years	Positive	No
Levin et al. (2008)	Cohort	64 smokers	6.4 years	Negative	Yes
Romanos et al. (2013)	Cohort	8 smokers	~5 years	Negative	Yes
Twito and Sade (2014)	Cohort	NA	6 years	Positive	No
Sun et al. (2016)	Cohort	16 smokers	1 year	Positive	No

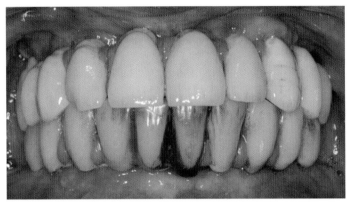

Surgical and Prosthetic Treatment: Dr. Georgios Romanos (Stony Brook, NY, USA)

Figure 21.19 Clinical photograph of a smoker with immediate loading in the maxilla and mandible eight years after treatment.

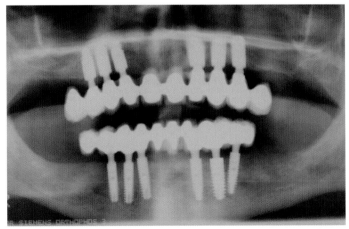

Surgical and Prosthetic Treatment: Dr. Georgios Romanos (Stony Brook, NY, USA)

Figure 21.20 Radiographical demonstration of a heavy smoker eight years after treatment with immediate loading in the maxilla and mandible.

Table 21.2 Studies assessing the effect of waterpipe smoking on the success and survival of dental implants.

Peri-implant status in waterpipe smokers

Study/Reference	Study design	Outcome of study

> **No studies in indexed literature**

Maziak et al., 2015; Javed et al., 2016). However, WS has gained popularity in many Western countries such as Australia, Canada, United Kingdom, and the United States, particularly among the young individuals (Jawad et al., 2013; Primack et al., 2013; Vanderhoek et al., 2013; Carroll et al., 2014; Grant et al., 2014; Kassim et al., 2014). Waterpipe smokers often consider WS as less harmful than traditional cigarette smoking, as the tobacco smoke in waterpipes gets filtered through water, which absorbs nicotine. Moreover, many individuals start WS in an attempt to quit cigarette smoking (Shaikh et al., 2008). The prevalence of systemic conditions such as hypertension, tachycardia, and oxidative stress has been reported to be higher in waterpipe smokers than nonsmokers (Hakim et al., 2011; Nemmar et al., 2015). WS has also been associated with the development of lung cancer (Chaouachi and Sajid, 2010). Studies (Natto et al., 2004; Al-Amad et al., 2014; Javed et al., 2016; Waziry et al., 2016) have shown that similar to cigarette smoking, WS is also a risk factor for oral cancer, periodontal disease, and alveolar bone loss. One explanation for this is that WS and cigarettes expose their consumers to the same chemicals, such as nicotine, tar, oxidants, polyaromatic hydrocarbons, and carbon monoxide (Monzer et al., 2008; Aboaziza and Eissenberg, 2015). There is a possibility that the nicotine and chemicals associated with WS induce a state of oxidative stress in peri-implant tissues (gingiva and alveolar bone), thereby increasing the likelihood of peri-implant diseases via inflammatory response, and if left uncontrolled, implant failure/loss. It is therefore hypothesized that WS is a significant risk factor for peri-implant diseases; and peri-implant bleeding on probing, probing depth, and marginal bone loss are higher among cigar/pipe smokers compared with nonsmokers. However, to date there are no studies in indexed literature that have assessed this hypothesis. It has also been stated that global attention against WS is needed and WS should not be considered an alternative and safe way of smoking (Bibars et al., 2015). There is a need for long-term prospective and retrospective clinical studies assessing the influence of WS on peri-implant inflammatory parameters (Table 21.2).

Pipe and Cigar Smoking

Pipe and cigar smoking habits are common in many parts of the world, including the United States, and the habit is particularly common among individuals belonging to

Table 21.3 Studies assessing the effect of vaping on the success and survival of dental implants.

Peri-implant status in vaping individuals		
Study/Reference	Study design	Outcome of study

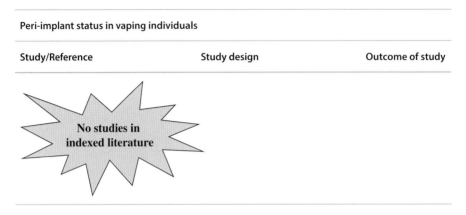

privileged socioeconomic groups (Kirkland, 1992; Gilpin et al., 1999; Kasza et al., 2017). The toxic constituents in cigar and pipe smoke are similar to those in cigarette smoke (Hecht, 2014; Chang et al., 2015); however, cigar smoke has been shown to have higher levels of tobacco-specific nitrosamines (TSNAs) than cigarette smoke due to the curing and fermentation process for cigar tobacco (Hecht, 2014; Chang et al., 2015). Wald and Watt (1997) suggested that cigarette smokers who have difficulty in quitting smoking may smoke cigars or pipes since the quantity of tobacco smoked and inhaled is less in cigar or pipe smoking compared with cigarette smoking. In the study by Feldman et al. (1983), calculus deposition, probing depth, and alveolar bone loss were significantly higher in cigarette smokers than pipe/cigar smokers. However, studies (Mulcahy, 1985; Chang et al., 2015) have also shown that cigar and pipe smoking is as hazardous to health as cigarettes.

Studies (Krall et al., 1999; Albandar et al., 2000) have shown that the prevalence of moderate and severe periodontitis is significantly higher in cigar and pipe smokers compared with nonsmokers. Albandar et al. (2000) predicted that the prevalence of moderate and severe periodontitis among cigar/pipe smokers is 17.6%. This study also showed that the number of site with clinical attachment loss ≥ 5 mm, probing depth ≥ 3 mm, and gingival recessions were significantly higher in cigar/pipe smokers compared with nonsmokers (Table 21.3).

Electronic Cigarette Smoking/Vaping

An electronic cigarette (e-cig) is a battery-operated device that consists of: (a) a metal heating element in a stainless-steel casing; (b) a container; (c) an atomizer; and (d) a battery. The container is filled with liquid, which usually contains nicotine, propylene glycol, glycerine, and artificial flavorings. A variety of aldehydes such as acrolein, acetaldehyde, and formaldehyde are present in the aerosols from e-cigs (Cheng, 2014; Kosmider et al., 2014). The heating device converts the liquid into vapor that is inhaled in the same manner as traditional tobacco smoking.

Individuals attempting to quit smoking believe that vaping e-cigs is an effective way to intake nicotine. Although studies demonstrating the detrimental effects of e-cig smoking on health are scare, experimental studies have shown that exposure to e-cig aerosols increases inflammatory and genotoxic stresses and induces DNA fragmentation in lung fibroblasts (Lerner et al., 2015; Lerner et al., 2016). In addition, increased production of destructive inflammatory cytokines (interleukin [IL]-6 and IL-8) in the lung fibroblasts has also been associated with vaping (Lerner et al., 2015; Lerner et al., 2016).

Interestingly, results from a recent in-vitro study (Sundar et al. 2016) showed that e-cigs with flavorings enhance oxidative stress and increase the release of destructive inflammatory cytokines (IL-8 and prostaglandin E2 [PGE2]) in human periodontal ligament fibroblasts, human gingival epithelium progenitors pooled, and epigingival 3D epithelium. In a pilot study, Wadia et al. (2016) compared the gingival status of smokers before and after substituting smoking tobacco with vaping. The results showed a significant increase in gingival inflammation when tobacco smokers switched to vaping from smoking (Wadia et al., 2016); however, these results should be interpreted with caution as they are based on a pilot study. Results from a recent review article suggested that vaping plays a role in the etiology of periodontal disease and oral premalignant lesions, such as oral submucous fibrosis (Javed et al., 2017). A proposed immuno-inflamamtory mechanism associated with peri-implant imflammation and bone loss in vaping individuals is shown in Figure 21.3. To our knowledge, there are no clinical studies assessing the effect of e-cig smoking on periodontal and peri-implant bone and soft-tissues. From the level of currently available experimental evidence, it seems that e-cig smoking may negatively influence the outcome of dentla implant therapy in a manner similar to conventional smoking by enhancing oxidative stress in periodontal and peri-implant tissues and augmenting alveolar bone loss. Hence, well-designed clinical studies are needed in this regard.

> ## Conclusion
>
> There is some evidence that dental implants can remain functionally stable in smokers. However, further studies are warranted in this regard.
>
> GRADE ACCORDING TO LEVEL OF EVIDENCE: **C**

References

Aboaziza, E. and Eissenberg, T. 2015. Waterpipe tobacco smoking: What is the evidence that it supports nicotine/tobacco dependence? *Tobacco Control* 24 Suppl 1, pp. i44–i53.

Al-Amad, S. H., Awad, M. A. and Nimri, O. 2014. Oral cancer in young Jordanians: Potential association with frequency of narghile smoking. *Oral Surgery, Oral Medicine, Oral Pathology, Oral Radiology, and Endodontology* 118, pp. 560–565.

Albandar, J. M., Streckfus, C. F., Adesanya, M. R. and Winn, D. M. 2000. Cigar, pipe, and cigarette smoking as risk factors for periodontal disease and tooth loss. *Journal of Periodontology* 71, pp. 1874–1881.

Almutairi, K. M. 2015. Predicting relationship of smoking behavior among male Saudi Arabian college students related to their religious practice. *Journal of Religion and Health* 10.1007/s10943-015-0003-z.

Aunmeungtong, W., Kumchai, T., Strietzel, F. P., Reichart, P. A. & Khongkhunthian, P. 2016. Comparative clinical study of conventional dental implants and mini dental implants for mandibular overdentures: A randomized clinical trial. *Clinical Implant Dentistry and Related Research* 10.1111/cid.12461.

Bain, C. A. and Moy, P. K. 1993. The association between the failure of dental implants and cigarette smoking. *The International Journal of Oral and Maxillofacial Implants* 8, pp. 609–615.

Balatsouka, D., Gotfredsen, K., Lindh, C. H. and Berglundh, T. 2005a. The impact of nicotine on bone healing and osseointegration. *Clinical Oral Implants Research* 16, pp. 268–276.

Balatsouka, D., Gotfredsen, K., Lindh, C. H. and Berglundh, T. 2005b. The impact of nicotine on osseointegration. An experimental study in the femur and tibia of rabbits. *Clinical Oral Implants Research* 16, pp. 389–395.

Berley, J., Yamano, S. and Sukotjo, C. 2010. The effect of systemic nicotine on osseointegration of titanium implants in the rat femur. *The Journal of Oral Implantology* 36, pp. 185–193.

Bibars, A. R., Obeidat, S. R., Khader, Y., Mahasneh, A. M. and Khabour, O. F. 2015. The effect of waterpipe smoking on periodontal health. *Oral Health and Preventive Dentistry* 13, pp. 253–259.

Borgan, S. M., Jassim, G., Marhoon, Z. A., Almuqamam, M. A., Ebrahim, M. A. and Soliman, P. A. 2014. Prevalence of tobacco smoking among health-care physicians in Bahrain. *BMC Public Health* 14, pp. 931.

Calvo-Guirado, J. L., Gomez-Moreno, G., Aguilar-Salvatierra, A., Guardia, J., Delgado-Ruiz, R. A. and Romanos, G. E. 2015. Marginal bone loss evaluation around immediate non-occlusal microthreaded implants placed in fresh extraction sockets in the maxilla: A 3-year study. *Clinical Oral Implants Research* 26, pp. 761–767.

Carroll, M. V., Chang, J., Sidani, J. E., Barnett, T. E., Soule, E., Balbach, E. and Primack, B. A. 2014. Reigniting tobacco ritual: Waterpipe tobacco smoking establishment culture in the United States. *Nicotine & Tobacco Research: Official Journal of the Society for Research on Nicotine and Tobacco* 16, pp. 1549–1558.

Cesar-Neto, J. B., Duarte, P. M., Sallum, E. A., Barbieri, D., Moreno, H., Jr. and Nociti, F. H., Jr. 2003. A comparative study on the effect of nicotine administration and cigarette smoke inhalation on bone healing around titanium implants. *Journal of Periodontology* 74, pp. 1454–1459.

Chang, C. M., Corey, C. G., Rostron, B. L. and Apelberg, B. J. 2015. Systematic review of cigar smoking and all cause and smoking related mortality. *BMC Public Health* 15, pp. 390.

Chaouachi, K. and Sajid, K. M. 2010. A critique of recent hypotheses on oral (and lung) cancer induced by water pipe (hookah, shisha, narghile) tobacco smoking. *Medical Hypotheses* 74, pp. 843–846.

Cheng, T. (2014). Chemical evaluation of electronic cigarettes. *Tobacco Control* 23 Suppl 2, pp. ii11–17.

Chrcanovic, B. R., Kisch, J., Albrektsson, T. and Wennerberg, A. 2016. Factors influencing early dental implant failures. *Journal of Dental Research* 95, pp. 995–1002.

Feldman, R. S., Bravacos, J. S. and Rose, C. L. 1983. Association between smoking different tobacco products and periodontal disease indexes. *Journal of Periodontology* 54, pp. 481–487.

Gilpin, E. A. and Pierce, J. P. 1999. Cigar smoking in California: 1990–1996. *American Journal of Preventive Medicine* 16, pp. 195–201.

Gotfredsen, K., Lindh, C. H. and Berglundh, T. 2009. Does longstanding nicotine exposure impair bone healing and osseointegration? An experimental study in rabbits. *Journal of Biomedical Materials Research. Part B: Applied Biomaterials* 91, pp. 918–923.

Grant, A., Morrison, R. and Dockrell, M. J. 2014. Prevalence of waterpipe (shisha, narghille, hookah) use among adults in Great Britain and factors associated with waterpipe use: Data from cross-sectional online surveys in 2012 and 2013. *Nicotine & Tobacco Research: Official Journal of the Society for Research on Nicotine and Tobacco* 16, pp. 931–938.

Hakim, F., Hellou, E., Goldbart, A., Katz, R., Bentur, Y. and Bentur, L. 2011. The acute effects of water-pipe smoking on the cardiorespiratory system. *Chest* 139, pp. 775–781.

Hecht, S. S. 2014. It is time to regulate carcinogenic tobacco-specific nitrosamines in cigarette tobacco. *Cancer Prevention Research (Philadelphia, Pa.)* 7, pp. 639–647.

Hoffmann, D. & Hoffmann, I. 1997. The changing cigarette, 1950–1995. *Journal of Toxicology and Environmental Health* 50, pp. 307–364.

Javed, F., Al-Kheraif, A. A., Rahman, I., Millan-Luongo, L. T., Feng, C., Yunker, M., Malmstrom, H. and Romanos, G. E. 2016. Comparison of clinical and radiographic periodontal status between habitual water-pipe smokers and cigarette smokers. *Journal of Periodontology* 87, pp. 142–147.

Javed, F., Kellesarian, S. V., Sundar, I. K., Romanos, G. E. and Rahman, I. 2017. Recent updates on electronic cigarette aerosol and inhaled nicotine effects on periodontal and pulmonary tissues. *Oral Diseases* 10.1111/odi.12652.

Javed, F. and Romanos, G. E. 2009. Impact of diabetes mellitus and glycemic control on the osseointegration of dental implants: A systematic literature review. *Journal of Periodontology* 80, pp. 1719–1730.

Jawad, M., Abass, J., Hariri, A., Rajasooriar, K. G., Salmasi, H., Millett, C. and Hamilton, F. L. 2013. Waterpipe smoking: Prevalence and attitudes among medical students in london. *The International Journal of Tuberculosis and Lung Disease: The Official Journal of the International Union against Tuberculosis and Lung Disease* 17, pp. 137–140.

Jawad, M., Nakkash, R. T., Mahfoud, Z., Bteddini, D., Haddad, P. and Afifi, R. A. 2015. Parental smoking and exposure to environmental tobacco smoke are associated with waterpipe smoking among youth: Results from a national survey in lebanon. *Public Health* 10.1016/j. puhe.2015.01.011.

Kassim, S., Al-Bakri, A., Al'Absi, M. and Croucher, R. 2014. Waterpipe tobacco dependence in U.K. Male adult residents: A cross-sectional study. *Nicotine & Tobacco Research: Official Journal of the Society for Research on Nicotine and Tobacco* 16, pp. 316–325.

Kasza, K. A., Ambrose, B. K., Conway, K. P., Borek, N., Taylor, K., Goniewicz, M. L., Cummings, K. M., Sharma, E., Pearson, J. L., Green, V. R., Kaufman, A. R., Bansal-Travers, M., Travers, M. J., Kwan, J., Tworek, C., Cheng, Y. C., Yang, L., Pharris-Ciurej, N., van Bemmel, D. M., Backinger, C. L., Compton, W. M. and Hyland, A. J. 2017. Tobacco-product use by adults and youths in the united states in 2013 and 2014. *The New England Journal of Medicine* 376, pp. 342–353.

Keenan, J. R. and Veitz-Keenan, A. 2016. The impact of smoking on failure rates, postoperative infection and marginal bone loss of dental implants. *Evidence-Based Dentistry* 17, pp. 4–5.

Kirkland, L. R. 1992. Bury me as a pipe smoker. *JAMA* 267, pp. 1073–1074.

Kosmider, L., Sobczak, A., Fik, M., Knysak, J., Zaciera, M., Kurek, J. and Goniewicz, M. L. 2014. Carbonyl compounds in electronic cigarette vapors: Effects of nicotine solvent and battery output voltage. *Nicotine & Tobacco Research: Official Journal of the Society for Research on Nicotine and Tobacco* 16, pp. 1319–1326.

Krall, E. A., Garvey, A. J. and Garcia, R. I. 1999. Alveolar bone loss and tooth loss in male cigar and pipe smokers. *Journal of the American Dental Association (1939)* 130, pp. 57–64.

Lerner, C. A., Rutagarama, P., Ahmad, T., Sundar, I. K., Elder, A. and Rahman, I. 2016. Electronic cigarette aerosols and copper nanoparticles induce mitochondrial stress and promote DNA fragmentation in lung fibroblasts. *Biochemical and Biophysical Research Communications* 477, pp. 620–625.

Lerner, C. A., Sundar, I. K., Yao, H., Gerloff, J., Ossip, D. J., McIntosh, S., Robinson, R. and Rahman, I. 2015. Vapors produced by electronic cigarettes and e-juices with flavorings induce toxicity, oxidative stress, and inflammatory response in lung epithelial cells and in mouse lung. *PloS One* 10, pp. e0116732.

Levin, L., Hertzberg, R., Har-Nes, S. and Schwartz-Arad, D. 2008. Long-term marginal bone loss around single dental implants affected by current and past smoking habits. *Implant Dentistry* 17, pp. 422–429.

Maziak, W., Taleb, Z. B., Bahelah, R., Islam, F., Jaber, R., Auf, R. and Salloum, R. G. 2015. The global epidemiology of waterpipe smoking. *Tobacco Control* 24, pp. i3–i12.

Moh'd Al-Mulla, A., Abdou Helmy, S., Al-Lawati, J., Al Nasser, S., Ali Abdel Rahman, S., Almutawa, A., Abi Saab, B., Al-Bedah, A. M., Al-Rabeah, A. M., Ali Bahaj, A., El-Awa, F., Warren, C. W., Jones, N. R. & Asma, S. 2008. Prevalence of tobacco use among students aged 13–15 years in health ministers' council/gulf cooperation council member states, 2001–2004. *The Journal of School Health* 78, pp. 337–343.

Monzer, B., Sepetdjian, E., Saliba, N. and Shihadeh, A. (2008). Charcoal emissions as a source of co and carcinogenic pah in mainstream narghile waterpipe smoke. *Food and Chemical Toxicology: An International Journal Published for the British Industrial Biological Research Association* 46, pp. 2991–2995.

Mulcahy, R. 1985. Cigar and pipe smoking and the heart. *British Medical Journal (Clinical Research ed.)* 290, pp. 951–952.

Natto, S., Baljoon, M., Abanmy, A. and Bergstrom, J. 2004. Tobacco smoking and gingival health in a Saudi Arabian population. *Oral Health & Preventive Dentistry* 2, pp. 351–357.

Natto, S. B. 2005. Tobacco smoking and periodontal health in a Saudi Arabian population. *Swedish Dental Journal. Supplement*, pp. 8–52, table of contents.

Nemmar, A., Yuvaraju, P., Beegam, S. and Ali, B. H. 2015. Short-term nose-only water-pipe (shisha) smoking exposure accelerates coagulation and causes cardiac inflammation and oxidative stress in mice. *Cellular Physiology and Biochemistry: International Journal of Experimental Cellular Physiology, Biochemistry, and Pharmacology* 35, pp. 829–840.

Primack, B. A., Shensa, A., Kim, K. H., Carroll, M. V., Hoban, M. T., Leino, E. V., Eissenberg, T., Dachille, K. H. and Fine, M. J. 2013. Waterpipe smoking among u.S. University students. *Nicotine & Tobacco Research : Official Journal of the Society for Research on Nicotine and Tobacco* 15, pp. 29–35.

Romanos, G. E., Gaertner, K., Aydin, E. and Nentwig, G. H. 2013. Long-term results after immediate loading of platform-switched implants in smokers versus nonsmokers with full-arch restorations. *The International Journal of Oral & Maxillofacial Implants* 28, pp. 841–845.

Romanos, G. E., Gaertner, K. and Nentwig, G. H. 2014. Long-term evaluation of immediately loaded implants in the edentulous mandible using fixed bridges and platform shifting. *Clinical Implant Dentistry and Related Research* 16, pp. 601–608.

Romanos, G. E., Javed, F., Delgado-Ruiz, R. A. and Calvo-Guirado, J. L. 2015. Peri-implant diseases: A review of treatment interventions. *Dental Clinics of North America* 59, pp. 157–178.

Romich, J. A. 2005. Fundamentals of pharmacology for veterinary technicians: Thomson Delmar Learning.

Rosa, G. M., Lucas, G. Q. and Lucas, O. N. 2008. Cigarette smoking and alveolar bone in young adults: A study using digitized radiographs. *Journal of Periodontology* 79, pp. 232–244.

Saaby, M., Karring, E., Schou, S. and Isidor, F. 2016. Factors influencing severity of peri-implantitis. *Clinical Oral Implants Research* 27, pp. 7–12.

Shaikh, R. B., Vijayaraghavan, N., Sulaiman, A. S., Kazi, S. and Shafi, M. S. 2008. The acute effects of waterpipe smoking on the cardiovascular and respiratory systems. *Journal of Preventive Medicine and Hygiene* 49, pp. 101–107.

Soares, E. V., Favaro, W. J., Cagnon, V. H., Bertran, C. A. and Camilli, J. A. 2010. Effects of alcohol and nicotine on the mechanical resistance of bone and bone neoformation around hydroxyapatite implants. *Journal of Bone and Mineral Metabolism* 28, pp. 101–107.

Stefani, C. M., Nogueira, F., Sallum, E. A., de, T. S., Sallum, A. W. and Nociti, F. H., Jr. 2002. Influence of nicotine administration on different implant surfaces: A histometric study in rabbits. *Journal of Periodontology* 73, pp. 206–212.

Sun, C., Zhao, J., Jianghao, C. and Hong, T. 2016. Effect of heavy smoking on dental implants placed in male patients posterior mandibles: A prospective clinical study. *The Journal of Oral Implantology* 42, pp. 477–483.

Sundar, I. K., Javed, F., Romanos, G. E. and Rahman, I. 2016. E-cigarettes and flavorings induce inflammatory and pro-senescence responses in oral epithelial cells and periodontal fibroblasts. *Oncotarget* 7, pp. 77196–77204.

Twito, D. and Sade, P. 2014. The effect of cigarette smoking habits on the outcome of dental implant treatment. *PeerJ* 2, pp. e546.

Vanderhoek, A. J., Hammal, F., Chappell, A., Wild, T. C., Raupach, T. and Finegan, B. A. 2013. Future physicians and tobacco: An online survey of the habits, beliefs and knowledge base of medical students at a Canadian university. *Tobacco Induced Diseases* 11, pp. 9.

Vervaeke, S., Collaert, B., Vandeweghe, S., Cosyn, J., Deschepper, E. and De Bruyn, H. 2012. The effect of smoking on survival and bone loss of implants with a fluoride-modified surface: A 2-year retrospective analysis of 1106 implants placed in daily practice. *Clinical Oral Implants Research* 23, pp. 758–766.

Wadia, R., Booth, V., Yap, H. F. and Moyes, D. L. 2016. A pilot study of the gingival response when smokers switch from smoking to vaping. *British Dental Journal* 221, pp. 722–726.

Wald, N. J. and Watt, H. C. 1997. Prospective study of effect of switching from cigarettes to pipes or cigars on mortality from three smoking related diseases. *BMJ (Clinical Research Ed.)* 314, pp. 1860–1863.

Wallace, R. H. 2000. The relationship between cigarette smoking and dental implant failure. *The European Journal of Prosthodontics and Restorative Dentistry* 8, pp. 103–106.

Waziry, R., Jawad, M., Ballout, R. A., Al Akel, M. and Akl, E. A. 2016. The effects of waterpipe tobacco smoking on health outcomes: An updated systematic review and meta-analysis. *International Journal of Epidemiology* 10.1093/ije/dyw021.

Yamano, S., Berley, J. A., Kuo, W. P., Gallucci, G. O., Weber, H. P. and Sukotjo, C. 2010. Effects of nicotine on gene expression and osseointegration in rats. *Clinical Oral Implants Research* 21, pp. 1353–1359.

22

Dental Implants in Patients with Genetic Disorders

Introduction

The building blocks of heredity are genes, which are passed from parent to child. These genes hold DNA, the instructions for making proteins. In humans, genes vary in size from a few hundred DNA bases to more than 2 million bases. Mutations in genes can expose an individual to a medical condition called *genetic disorder*. Most genetic disorders are quite rare and affect one person in every several thousands or millions. There are three types of genetic disorders:

1) Single-gene disorders, where a mutation affects one gene. An example in this regard is sickle cell anemia.
2) Chromosomal disorders, where chromosomes (or parts of chromosomes) are missing or changed. Down syndrome (DS) is a classic example of a chromosomal disorder.
3) Complex disorders, where there are mutations in two or more genes. Colon cancer is an example.

Dental Implants in Patients with Genetic Disorders

Down Syndrome

DS, also known as trisomy 21, is an autosomal chromosomal anomaly that occurs mostly due to carrying an extra chromosome 21 (Delabar et al., 1993). In the United States, approximately 14.47 per 10,000 live births occur with DS (Parker et al., 2010). The most common dentofacial manifestations among patients with DS include a high incidence of dental caries, hypodontia, a compromised occlusal vertical dimension, periodontal disease, tooth structure anomalies, malocclusion, tooth wear due to bruxism, hypotonic orofacial musculature, and xerostomia (Scully, 1976; Desai, 1997; Hennequin et al., 1999; Seagriff-Curtin et al., 2006; Horbelt, 2007; Mehr et al., 2015; Tanaka et al., 2015; Martins et al., 2016; Mubayrik, 2016). Moreover, skeletal defects such as an underdeveloped maxillary arch and mandibular prognathism are also common manifestations in patients with DS (Suri et al., 2010; Silva Jesuino and Valladares-Neto, 2013; Rey et al., 2015).

A limited number of studies (mainly case-reports) have assessed the outcome of dental implant therapy among patients with DS (Lustig et al., 2002; Soares et al., 2010; Ribeiro et al., 2011; Ekfeldt et al., 2013; Limeres Posse et al., 2016; Saponaro et al., 2016; Alqahtani et al., 2017; Altintas et al., 2017; Corcuera-Flores et al., 2017) (Table 22.1).

Evidence-based Implant Dentistry and Systemic Conditions, First Edition.
Fawad Javed and Georgios E. Romanos.
© 2018 John Wiley & Sons, Inc. Published 2018 by John Wiley & Sons, Inc.

Table 22.1 Outcomes of studies assessing the success and survival of dental implants in patients with Down syndrome.

Authors et al. (Year)	Study design	Participant/s	Implant therapy	Follow-up	Peri-implant status at follow-up
Lustig et al. (2002)	Case-report	16-year-old male	Implant placed in the area of missing maxillary left and right premolars and mandibular right premolar	2.5 years	The implants were stable and the prosthesis was functioning well.
Soares et al. (2010)	Case-report	22-year-old male	Implant placed in the area of missing maxillary left central incisor	4-years	The implant was stable at follow-up.
Ribeiro et al. (2011)	Case-report	36-year-old female	Maxillary and mandibular implant-retained overdenture prosthesis	2.3 years	The implants were stable and the prosthesis was functioning well.
Ekfeldt et al. (2013)	Prospective	Patient 1: 48-year-old male Patient 2: 46-year-old female Patient 3: 54-year-old male Patient 4: 19-year-old male	Implants placed in the right mandibular quadrant Implant placed in the area of missing maxillary left central incisor Implant placed in the area of missing maxillary right central incisor Implant placed in the area of missing maxillary right and left canines	6 years 9 years NA 6.5 years	Three out of the four implants placed in DS patients failed.
Limeres Posse et al. (2016)	Retrospective	NA: At least 18 years old	Maxilla and mandible*	1 year	The success rate for dental implants in individuals with Down syndrome seems to be lower than that observed in the general population.
Saponaro et al. (2016)	Case-report	27-year-old female	Mandibular implant-retained fixed prosthesis	1.8 years	The implants were stable and the prosthesis was functioning well.
Alqahtani et al. (2017)	Case-report	44-year-old male	Immediate implant placed in the area of missing maxillary left central incisor	6 months	Not reported
Altintas et al. (2017)	Case-report	37-year-old female	Maxillary and mandibular implant-retained overdenture prosthesis	2 years	The implants were stable and the prosthesis was functioning well.
Corcuera-Flores et al. (2017)	Retrospective	19 DS patients and 22 controls	102 dental implants were placed in DS patients and 70 implants in healthy controls.	4 years	Peri-implant marginal bone loss was significantly higher in DS patients than controls.

DS: Down's syndrome
NA: Not available
*Implant location was unclear

Results, from nearly 50% of the studies, showed that dental implants can osseointegrate and remain functionally stable in patients with DS. However, these results should be interpreted with caution as the outcomes were based on mostly case-reports. Clenching habits, tongue pressure, and changes in proprioception are possible factors that may jeopardize osseointegration and success/survival of dental implants in the patients with DS. It is highly recommended that patients with DS and their caretakers should be educated about significance of routine oral hygiene maintenance that may play a role in the long-term success and survival of dental implants in DS patients (Figures 22.1 to 22.3).

Figure 22.1a Implant-retained telescopic prosthesis in the mandible for a patient with Down syndrome.

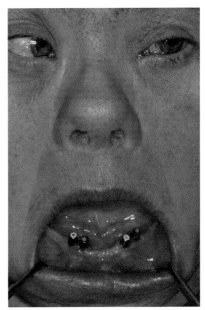

Surgical and prosthetic treatment: Dr. D. May (Luenen, Germany)

Figure 22.1b The prosthesis in place.

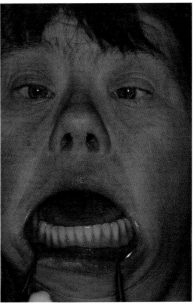

Surgical and prosthetic treatment: Dr. D. May (Luenen, Germany)

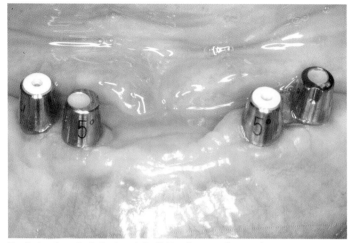

Surgical and prosthetic treatment: Dr. D. May (Luenen, Germany)

Figure 22.2 Clinical situation: 5 years of loading.

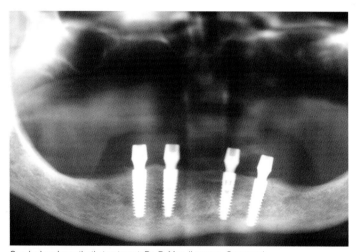

Surgical and prosthetic treatment: Dr. D. May (Luenen, Germany)

Figure 22.3 Radiographic evaluation five years after treatment shows crestal bone stability.

Huntington's Disease

Huntington's disease (HD) is an adult-onset, autosomal dominant, and incurable inherited genetic disorder associated with mutations in the Huntingtin (HTT) gene and cell loss within a specific subset of neurons in the basal ganglia and cortex (Wiatr et al., 2017). Characteristic features of HD include behavioral changes, dementia, and involuntary movements (Deniz et al., 2011). Symptom onset usually occurs by the age of 40 years, but this can be very variable. The age of HD onset is related to the size of the mutation. Compared to healthy individuals, patients with HD show significantly more dental caries and plaque accumulation on teeth (Saft et al., 2013).

Table 22.2 Characteristics and outcome of the study that assessed osseointegration and survival of dental implants in patients with Huntington's disease.

Authors et al. (Year)	Study design	Participant/s	Implant therapy	Follow-up	Peri-implant status at follow-up
Jackowski et al. (2001)	Case-report	56-year-old male	Implant supported mandibular over-denture.	1-year	The implants were stable and the prosthesis was functioning well.
Deniz et al. (2011)	Case-report	67-year-old female	Implant supported mandibular over-denture.	1-year	The implants were stable and the prosthesis was functioning well.

To date, only two case-reports have assessed the outcome of dental implant therapy among patients with Huntington's disease (Jackowski et al., 2001; Deniz et al., 2011) (Table 22.2). In each of these case-reports, implant-supported mandibular overdentures were provided to patients with HD. One-year follow-up results showed that dental implants had osseointegrated and the dental prostheses were functional. However, these outcomes should be interpreted with extreme caution, as they were based merely on case-reports and the follow-up duration of each case-report was short (12 months).

Conclusion
There is insufficient evidence to determine whether dental implants can osseointegrate and remain functionally stable among patients with genetic disorders
GRADE ACCORDING TO LEVEL OF EVIDENCE: **D**

References

Alqahtani, N. M., Alsayed, H. D., Levon, J. A. and Brown, D. T. 2017. Prosthodontic rehabilitation for a patient with Down syndrome: a clinical report. *Journal of Prosthodontics*. doi:10.1111/jopr.12595.

Altintas, N. Y., Kilic, S. and Altintas, S. H. 2017. Oral rehabilitation with implant-retained overdenture in a patient with Down syndrome. *Journal of Prosthodontics*. doi:10.1111/jopr.12596.

Corcuera-Flores, J. R., Lopez-Gimenez, J., Lopez-Jimenez, J., Lopez-Gimenez, A., Silvestre-Rangil, J. and Machuca-Portillo, G. 2017. Four years survival and marginal bone loss of implants in patients with Down syndrome and cerebral palsy. *Clinical Oral Investigations* 21, pp. 1667–1674. doi:10.1007/s00784-016-1970-5.

Delabar, J. M., Theophile, D., Rahmani, Z., Chettouh, Z., Blouin, J. L., Prieur, M., Noel, B. and Sinet, P. M. 1993. Molecular mapping of twenty-four features of Down syndrome on chromosome 21. *European Journal of Human Genetics* 1, pp. 114–124.

Deniz, E., Kokat, A. M. and Noyan, A. 2011. Implant-supported overdenture in an elderly patient with Huntington's disease. *Gerodontology* 28, pp. 157–160. doi:10.1111/j.1741-2358.2009.00343.x.

Desai, S. S. 1997. Down syndrome: a review of the literature. *Oral Surgery, Oral Medicine, Oral Pathology, Oral Radiology, and Endodontology* 84, pp. 279–285.

Ekfeldt, A., Zellmer, M. and Carlsson, G. E. 2013. Treatment with implant-supported fixed dental prostheses in patients with congenital and acquired neurologic disabilities: a prospective study. *International Journal of Prosthodontics* 26, pp. 517–524. doi:10.11607/ijp.3511.

Hennequin, M., Faulks, D., Veyrune, J. L. and Bourdiol, P. 1999. Significance of oral health in persons with Down syndrome: a literature review. *Devopmental Medicine and Child Neurology* 41, pp. 275–283.

Horbelt, C. V. (2007). Down syndrome: a review of common physical and oral characteristics. *General Dentistry* 55, 399–402.

Jackowski, J., Andrich, J., Kappeler, H., Zollner, A., Johren, P. and Muller, T. 2001. Implant-supported denture in a patient with Huntington's disease: interdisciplinary aspects. *Spec Care Dentist* 21, pp. 15–20.

Limeres Posse, J., Lopez Jimenez, J., Ruiz Villandiego, J. C., Cutando Soriano, A., Fernandez Feijoo, J., Linazasoro Elorza, M., Diniz Freitas, M. and Diz Dios, P. 2016. Survival of dental implants in patients with Down syndrome: A case series. *Journal of Prosthetics Dentistry* 116, pp. 880–884. doi:10.1016/j.prosdent.2016.04.015.

Lustig, J. P., Yanko, R. and Zilberman, U. 2002. Use of dental implants in patients with Down syndrome: a case report. *Special Care Dentistry Association* 22, pp. 201–204.

Martins, F., Simoes, A., Oliveira, M., Luiz, A. C., Gallottini, M. and Pannuti, C. 2016. Efficacy of antimicrobial photodynamic therapy as an adjuvant in periodontal treatment in Down syndrome patients. *Lasers in Medical Science* 31, pp. 1977–1981. doi:10.1007/s10103-016-2020-x.

Mehr, A. K., Zarandi, A. and Anush, K. 2015. Prevalence of oral trichomonas tenax in periodontal lesions of Down syndrome in Tabriz, Iran. *Journal of Clinical Diagnosis Res* 9, pp. Zc88–90. doi:10.7860/jcdr/2015/14725.6238.

Mubayrik, A. B. 2016. The dental needs and treatment of patients with Down syndrome. *Dental Clinics of North America* 60, pp. 613–626. doi:10.1016/j.cden.2016.02.003.

Parker, S. E., Mai, C. T., Canfield, M. A., Rickard, R., Wang, Y., Meyer, R. E., Anderson, P., Mason, C. A., Collins, J. S., Kirby, R. S. and Correa, A. 2010. Updated national birth prevalence estimates for selected birth defects in the United States, 2004–2006. *Birth Defects Research, Part A: Clinical Molecular Teratology* 88, pp. 1008–1016. doi:10.1002/bdra.20735.

Rey, D., Campuzano, A. and Ngan, P. 2015. Modified Alt-RAMEC treatment of Class III malocclusion in young patients with Down syndrome. *Journal of Clinical Orthodontics* 49, pp. 113–120.

Ribeiro, C. G., Siqueira, A. F., Bez, L., Cardoso, A. C. and Ferreira, C. F. 2011. Dental implant rehabilitation of a patient with down syndrome: a case report. *Journal of Oral Implantology* 37, pp. 481–487. doi:10.1563/aaid-joi-d-10-00003.1.

Saft, C., Andrich, J. E., Muller, T., Becker, J. and Jackowski, J. 2013. Oral and dental health in Huntington's disease – an observational study. *BMC Neurology* 13, pp. 114. doi:10.1186/1471-2377-13-114.

Saponaro, P. C., Deguchi, T. and Lee, D. J. 2016. Implant therapy for a patient with Down syndrome and oral habits: A clinical report. *Journal of Prosthetic Dentistry* 116, pp. 320–324. doi:10.1016/j.prosdent.2016.01.019.

Scully, C. 1976. Down's syndrome: aspects of dental care. *Journal of Dentistry* 4, pp. 167–174.

Seagriff-Curtin, P., Pugliese, S. and Romer, M. 2006. Dental considerations for individuals with Down syndrome. *New York State Dental Journal* 72, pp. 33–35.

Silva Jesuino, F. A. and Valladares-Neto, J. 2013. Craniofacial morphological differences between Down syndrome and maxillary deficiency children. *European Journal of Orthodontics* 35, pp. 124–130. doi:10.1093/ejo/cjr105.

Soares, M. R., de Paula, F. O., Chaves, M., Assis, N. M. and Chaves Filho, H. D. 2010. Patient with Down syndrome and implant therapy: a case report. *Brazilian Dental Journal* 21, 550–554.

Suri, S., Tompson, B. D. and Cornfoot, L. 2010. Cranial base, maxillary and mandibular morphology in Down syndrome. *Angle Orthodontist* 80, pp. 861–869. doi:10.2319/111709-650.1.

Tanaka, M. H., Rodrigues, T. O., Finoti, L. S., Teixeira, S. R., Mayer, M. P., Scarel-Caminaga, R. M. and Giro, E. M. 2015. The effect of conventional mechanical periodontal treatment on red complex microorganisms and clinical parameters in Down syndrome periodontitis patients: a pilot study. *European Journal of Clinical Microbiology and Infectious Diseases* 34, pp. 601–608. doi:10.1007/s10096-014-2268-7.

Wiatr, K., Szlachcic, W. J., Trzeciak, M., Figlerowicz, M. and Figiel, M. 2017. Huntington Disease as a neurodevelopmental disorder and early signs of the disease in stem cells. *Molecular Neurobiology*. doi:10.1007/s12035-017-0477-7.

23

Dental Implants in Patients with Human Immunodeficiency Virus Infection or Acquired Immune Deficiency Syndrome

Introduction

Periodontal Health Status among Patients with HIV and AIDS Infections

Studies have shown that periodontal health status is compromised among patients infected with the human immunodeficiency virus (HIV) and acquired immune deficiency syndrome (AIDS) (Myint et al., 2002; Nouaman et al., 2015; Frimpong et al., 2017). However, results from a recent cohort study showed no statistically significant difference in periodontal diseases among the HIV-infected and noninfected individuals after the data was adjusted for plaque control habits and behavioral and socio-demographic factors (Ryder et al., 2017).

Impact of HIV Infection and AIDS on Osseointegration

In a monocentric study, 66 HIV-infected patients with a stable disease with good oral hygiene, requiring implant rehabilitation, were included (Gherlone et al., 2016a). In this study, each patient received at least one dental implant, with a total of 190 implants placed in the study population. The primary outcome variables were implant failure, prosthetic failure, peri-implant marginal bone loss, and biological complications, including peri-implantitis, pus discharge, pain, and paresthesia (Gherlone et al., 2016a). The peri-implant status was assessed at the time in intervention and after 12 months of follow-up.

At follow-up, there was no evidence of fractures of fixtures or paresthesia and implant failure occurred in patients (15 out of the 190 fixtures) (Gherlone et al., 2016a). The study concluded that dental implant therapy is a suitable therapeutic strategy for oral rehabilitation in HIV-infected patients provided the disease is well controlled and appropriate infection control protocols are adopted (Gherlone et al., 2016a). Similar results were reported in another study (Gherlone et al., 2016b) (Figures 23.1 to 23.7).

Objective

The aim of this chapter to review indexed literature to determine whether dental implants can remain functionally stable in patients with HIV infection and AIDS.

Evidence-based Implant Dentistry and Systemic Conditions, First Edition.
Fawad Javed and Georgios E. Romanos.
© 2018 John Wiley & Sons, Inc. Published 2018 by John Wiley & Sons, Inc.

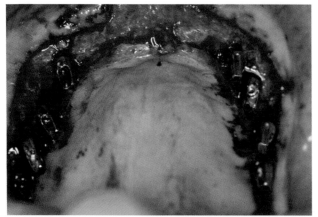

Surgical and Prosthetic Treatment: Dr. Georgios Romanos (Stony Brook, NY, USA)
Dental technician: L. Marotta (Marotta Dental Studio, Farmingdale, NY, USA)

Figure 23.1 Immediate loading in the maxilla of an HIV-positive patient. (*Source:* Romanos, 2012. Reproduced with permission of Quintessence).

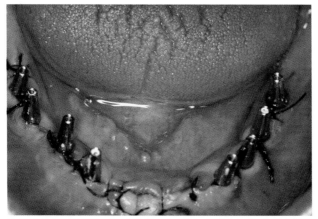

Surgical and Prosthetic Treatment: Dr. Georgios Romanos (Stony Brook, NY, USA)
Dental technician: L. Marotta (Marotta Dental Studio, Farmingdale, NY, USA)

Figure 23.2 Immediate loading in the mandible of an HIV-positive patient.

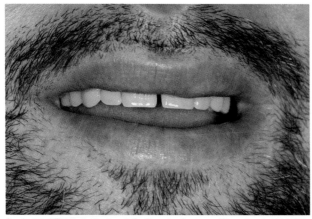

Surgical and Prosthetic Treatment: Dr. Georgios Romanos (Stony Brook, NY, USA)
Dental technician: L. Marotta (Marotta Dental Studio, Farmingdale, NY, USA)

Figure 23.3 Provisional restoration after surgery.

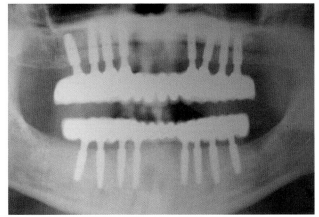

Surgical and Prosthetic Treatment: Dr. Georgios Romanos (Stony Brook, NY, USA)
Dental technician: L. Marotta (Marotta Dental Studio, Farmingdale, NY, USA)

Figure 23.4 Radiographic examination one year after surgery with the provisional prostheses in place. (*Source:* Romanos, 2012. Reproduced with permission of Quintessence).

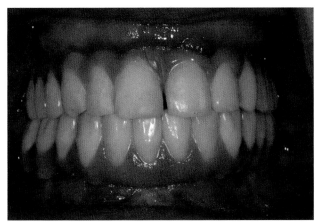

Surgical and Prosthetic Treatment: Dr. Georgios Romanos (Stony Brook, NY, USA)
Dental technician: L. Marotta (Marotta Dental Studio, Farmingdale, NY, USA)

Figure 23.5 Clinical evaluation 12 years after treatment.

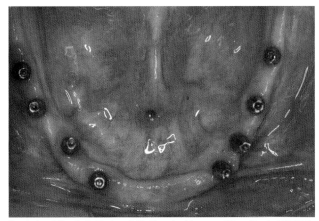

Surgical and Prosthetic Treatment: Dr. Georgios Romanos (Stony Brook, NY, USA)
Dental technician: L. Marotta (Marotta Dental Studio, Farmingdale, NY, USA)

Figure 23.6 Healthy peri-implant soft tissues 12 years after treatment in the mandibular arch.

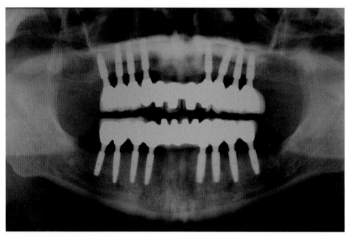

Surgical and Prosthetic Treatment: Dr. Georgios Romanos (Stony Brook, NY, USA)
Dental technician: L. Marotta (Marotta Dental Studio, Farmingdale, NY, USA)

Figure 23.7 Radiographic evaluation 12 years after treatment demonstrating slight crestal bone loss.

Materials and Methods

Eligibility Criteria

The following eligibility criteria were entailed: (a) clinical and experimental studies and (b) placement and survival of dental implants in animals or human patients with HIV infection or AIDS. Literature reviews, letters to the editor, and commentaries were excluded.

Literature Search

PubMed/Medline (National Library of Medicine, Bethesda, Maryland), EMBASE, ISI-Web of Knowledge, SCOPUS, and Google-Scholar databases were searched up to February 2018 using the following key words in different combinations: "human immunodeficiency virus," "dental implant," "failure," "HIV," "AIDS," "acquired immune deficiency syndrome," "survival," and "success." Titles and abstracts of studies that fulfilled the eligibility criteria were screened and checked for agreement. Full texts of studies judged by title and abstract to be relevant were read and assessed in accordance with the eligibility criteria (as already stated). In addition, hand searching of the reference lists of potentially relevant original and review studies was also performed and checked for agreement via discussion.

Results

In total, 13 studies were identified (Rajnay and Hochstetter, 1998; Baron et al., 2004; Achong et al., 2006; Strietzel et al., 2006; Stevenson et al., 2007; Kolhatkar et al., 2011; Oliveira et al., 2011; Romanos et al., 2014; Gay-Escoda et al., 2016; Gherlone et al., 2016a; Gherlone et al., 2016b; May et al., 2016; Vidal et al., 2017). The study participants ranged between 1 and 68 patients and the duration of follow-up ranged between 4 weeks and 10 years. Results from nearly 50% of the studies were based on case-reports and

Table 23.1 Outcomes of studies assessing the success and survival of dental implants in patients with HIV/AIDS.

Authors et al.	Study design	Participant/s	HIV/AIDS	Follow-up	Outcome
Rajnay and Hochstetter (1998)	Case-report	1 patient	HIV+	~1.5 years	Dental implants can remain functionally stable in HIV-positive patients with stable disease.
Baron et al. (2005)	Case-report	1 patient	HIV+	2 years	Dental implants can remain functionally stable in HIV-positive patients with stable disease.
Achong et al. (2006)	Case-series	3 patients	HIV+	2 years	Dental implants can remain functionally stable in HIV-positive patients with stable disease.
Strietzel et al. (2006)	Case-series	3 patients	HIV+	~3 years	Dental implants can remain functionally stable in HIV-positive patients with stable disease.
Stevenson et al. (2007)	Prospective	20 patients	HIV+	6 months	Dental implants can remain functionally stable in HIV-positive patients with stable disease.
Kolhatkar et al. (2011)	Retrospective	2 patients	HIV+	Up to 4 weeks	Dental implants can remain functionally stable in HIV-positive patients with stable disease.
Oliveira et al. (2011)	Prospective	40 patients	HIV+	1 year	Dental implants can remain functionally stable in HIV-positive patients with stable disease.
Romanos et al. (2014)	Case-report	43-year-old male	HIV+	4 years	Dental implants can remain functionally stable in HIV-positive patients with stable disease.
Gay-Escoda et al. (2016)	Case-series	9 patients	HIV+	~6 years	Dental implants can remain functionally stable in HIV-positive patients with stable disease.
Gherlone et al. (2016a)	Prospective	68 patients	HIV+	1 year	Dental implants can remain functionally stable in HIV-positive patients with stable disease.
Gherlone et al. (2016b)	Retrospective	66 patients	HIV+	1 year	Dental implants can remain functionally stable in HIV-positive patients with stable disease.
May et al. (2016)	Retrospective	16 patients	AIDS	5 years	Dental implants can remain functionally stable in HIV-positive patients with stable disease.
Vidal et al. (2017)	Case-series	3 patients	HIV+	Up to 10 years	Dental implants can remain functionally stable in HIV-positive patients with stable disease.

case-series (Rajnay and Hochstetter, 1998; Baron et al., 2004; Achong et al., 2006; Strietzel et al., 2006; Romanos et al., 2014; Gay-Escoda et al., 2016; Vidal et al., 2017). All studies reported that dental implants can remain functionally stable in HIV-positive patients with stable disease (Table 23.1).

Discussion

It is tempting to speculate that dental implants can osseointegrate and remain function-ally stable in HIV+ patients and individuals with AIDS; however, the outcomes of implant therapy as reported in this chapter should be interpreted with caution. This is primarily due to the fact that the level of evidence from nearly 50% of the studies was low, as the outcomes were based on case-reports and case-series (Rajnay and Hochstetter, 1998; Baron et al., 2004; Achong et al., 2006; Strietzel et al., 2006; Romanos et al., 2014; Gay-Escoda et al., 2016; Vidal et al., 2017). Moreover, the prospective and retrospective stud-ies with a comparatively larger sample size had follow-up durations of only 12 months.

Conclusion
There is insufficient evidence to determine whether, in the long-term, dental implants can remain functionally stable in HIV+ patients and patients with AIDS. Hence, further studies are warranted in this regard. GRADE ACCORDING TO LEVEL OF EVIDENCE: **D**

References

Achong, R. M., Shetty, K., Arribas, A. and Block, M. S. 2006. Implants in HIV-positive patients: 3 case reports. *Journal of Oral and Maxillofacial Surgery* 64, pp. 1199–1203. doi:10.1016/j.joms.2006.04.037.

Baron, M., Gritsch, F., Hansy, A. M. and Haas, R. 2004. Implants in an HIV-positive patient: a case report. *International Journal of Oral and Maxillofacial Implants* 19, pp. 425–430.

Frimpong, P., Amponsah, E. K., Abebrese, J. and Kim, S. M. 2017. Oral manifestations and their correlation to baseline CD4 count of HIV/AIDS patients in Ghana. *Journal of the Korean Association of Oral Maxillofacial Surgery* 43, pp. 29–36. doi:10.5125/jkaoms.2017.43.1.29.

Gay-Escoda, C., Perez-Alvarez, D., Camps-Font, O. and Figueiredo, R. 2016. Long-term outcomes of oral rehabilitation with dental implants in HIV-positive patients: A retrospective case series. *Medicina Oral Patologia Oral Y Cirugia Bucal* 21, pp. e385–391.

Gherlone, E. F., Cappare, P., Tecco, S., Polizzi, E., Pantaleo, G., Gastaldi, G. and Grusovin, M. G. 2016a. Implant prosthetic rehabilitation in controlled HIV-positive patients: a prospective longitudinal study with 1-year follow-up. *Clinical Implant Dentistry and Related Research* 18, pp. 725–734. doi:10.1111/cid.12353.

Gherlone, E. F., Cappare, P., Tecco, S., Polizzi, E., Pantaleo, G., Gastaldi, G. and Grusovin, M. G. 2016b. A prospective longitudinal study on implant prosthetic rehabilitation in controlled HIV-positive patients with 1-year follow-up: the role of CD4+ level, smoking habits, and oral hygiene. *Clinical Implant Dentistry and Related Research* 18, pp. 955–964. doi:10.1111/cid.12370.

Kolhatkar, S., Khalid, S., Rolecki, A., Bhola, M. and Winkler, J. R. 2011. Immediate dental implant placement in HIV-positive patients receiving highly active antiretroviral therapy: a report of two cases and a review of the literature of implants placed in HIV-positive individuals. *Journal of Periodontology* 82, pp. 505–511. doi:10.1902/jop.2010.100433.

May, M. C., Andrews, P. N., Daher, S. and Reebye, U. N. 2016. Prospective cohort study of dental implant success rate in patients with AIDS. *International Journal of Implant Dentistry* 2, pp. 20. doi:10.1186/s40729-016-0053-3.

Myint, M., Steinsvoll, S., Yuan, Z. N., Johne, B., Helgeland, K. and Schenck, K. 2002. Highly increased numbers of leukocytes in inflamed gingiva from patients with HIV infection. *Aids* 16, pp. 235–243.

Nouaman, M. N., Meless, D. G., Coffie, P. A., Arrive, E., Tchounga, B. K., Ekouevi, D. K., Anoma, C., Eholie, S. P., Dabis, F. and Jaquet, A. 2015. Oral health and HIV infection among female sex workers in Abidjan, Cote d'Ivoire. *BMC Oral Health* 15, pp. 154. doi:10.1186/s12903-015-0129-0.

Oliveira, M. A., Gallottini, M., Pallos, D., Maluf, P. S., Jablonka, F. and Ortega, K. L. 2011. The success of endosseous implants in human immunodeficiency virus-positive patients receiving antiretroviral therapy: a pilot study. *Journal of the American Dental Association* 142, pp. 1010–1016.

Rajnay, Z. W. and Hochstetter, R. L. 1998. Immediate placement of an endosseous root-form implant in an HIV-positive patient: report of a case. *Journal of Periodontology* 69, pp. 1167–1171. doi:10.1902/jop.1998.69.10.1167.

Romanos, G. E., Goldin, E., Marotta, L., Froum, S. and Tarnow, D. P. 2014. Immediate loading with fixed implant-supported restorations in an edentulous patient with an HIV infection: a case report. *Implant Dentistry* 23, pp. 8–12. doi:10.1097/ID.0b013e3182a62766.

Ryder, M. I., Yao, T. J., Russell, J. S., Moscicki, A. B. and Shiboski, C. H. 2017. Prevalence of periodontal diseases in a multicenter cohort of perinatally HIV-infected and HIV-exposed and uninfected youth. *Journal of Clinical Periodontology* 44, pp. 2–12. doi:10.1111/jcpe.12646.

Stevenson, G. C., Riano, P. C., Moretti, A. J., Nichols, C. M., Engelmeier, R. L. and Flaitz, C. M. 2007. Short-term success of osseointegrated dental implants in HIV-positive individuals: a prospective study. *Journal of Contemporary Dental Practices* 8, pp. 1–10.

Strietzel, F. P., Rothe, S., Reichart, P. A. and Schmidt-Westhausen, A. M. 2006. Implant-prosthetic treatment in HIV-infected patients receiving highly active antiretroviral therapy: report of cases. *The International Journal of Oral & Maxillofacial Implants* 21, pp. 951–956.

Vidal, F., Vidal, R., Bochnia, J., de Souza, R. C. and Goncalves, L. S. 2017. Dental implants and bone augmentation in HIV-infected patients under HAART: Case report and review of the literature. *Special Care Dentistry* 37, pp. 150–155. doi:10.1111/scd.12219.

Index

Evidence-based Implant Dentistry and Systemic Conditions, First Edition.
Fawad Javed and Georgios E. Romanos.
© 2018 John Wiley & Sons, Inc. Published 2018 by John Wiley & Sons, Inc.